# ETHICS

SECOND EDITION

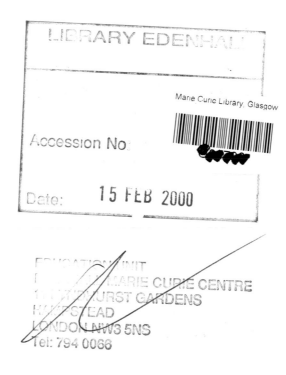

Education Department
Marie Curie Hospice
11 Lyndhurst Gardens
Hampstead, London NW3 5HS
Tel: 020 7853 3434
Fax: 020 7853 3436

FOR SIMON AND MARY ELSTOW

# ETHICS
# The Heart of Health Care

## SECOND EDITION

David Seedhouse
*University of Auckland, New Zealand*

**JOHN WILEY & SONS**
*Chichester · New York · Weinheim · Brisbane · Singapore · Toronto*

First published 1988
Reprinted 1989, 1991, 1992 (twice), 1993, 1994, 1995 and 1997
Second Edition 1998. Reprinted December 1998

*Other Wiley Editorial Offices*

John Wiley & Sons, Inc., 605 Third Avenue,
New York, NY 10158-0012, USA

WILEY-VCH Verlag GmbH, Pappelallee 3,
D-69469 Weinheim, Germany

Jacaranda Wiley Ltd, 33 Park Road, Milton,
Queensland 4064, Australia

John Wiley & Sons (Asia) Pte Ltd, 2 Clementi Loop #02-01,
Jin Xing Distripark, Singapore 129809

John Wiley & Sons (Canada) Ltd, 22 Worcester Road,
Rexdale, Ontario M9W 1L1, Canada

**Library of Congress Cataloging-in-Publication Data**

Seedhouse, David.
    Ethics : the heart of health care / David Seedhouse. – 2nd ed.
       p.   cm.
    Includes bibliographical references and index.
    ISBN 0-471-97592-3 (pbk.)
    1. Medical ethics.   I. Title.
    R724.S4325   1998                          97-46064
    174'.2 – dc21                               CIP

**British Library Cataloguing in Publication Data**

A catalogue record for this book is available from the British Library

ISBN 0-471-97592-3

# Contents

About the Author                                          vii

Preface                                                    ix

Preface to the First Edition                               xi

Acknowledgements                                           xv

Introduction                                                1

**PART ONE:       WORK FOR HEALTH IS A MORAL ENDEAVOUR**

Chapter One     Growing Pains                              23

Chapter Two     Ethics is the Key                          35

Chapter Three   Uncovering the Basic Questions             47

Chapter Four    Problems of Practice                       55

**PART TWO:       THE SEARCH FOR THE TRULY MORAL**

Chapter Five    The Search for Morality                    77

Chapter Six     What is a Person?                         105

Chapter Seven   Theories of Ethics                        113

Chapter Eight   Obstacles to Clear Moral Reasoning        135

**PART THREE: HOW TO MAKE ETHICALLY SOUND PRACTICAL
              DECISIONS**

Chapter Nine    The Rings of Uncertainty                  149

Chapter Ten     The Background to the Ethical Grid        177

Chapter Eleven  The Use of the Ethical Grid               211

References                                                221

Index                                                     225

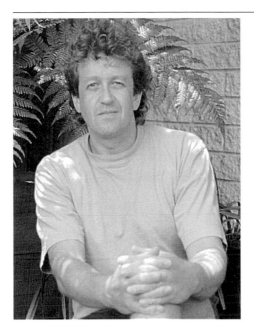

## ABOUT THE AUTHOR

**David Seedhouse** was born in Nottingham, England. He was educated at Carre's Grammar School, Sleaford (1967–74) and 'The Vic', Sleaford (1971–last orders). He continued this research programme at Manchester University (1977–84) and 'The Grafton', Rusholme (1977–?) where he achieved degrees in philosophy, and of memory loss.

Though captivated by good philosophical analysis and the prospect of uninterrupted lunch-time refreshment, David decided against a conventional academic career. He found most philosophy socially irrelevant (not least to fellow Graftonites) and determined to apply his philosophical skills to actual problems – not hypothetical ones.

To this end David accepted posts in health studies, nursing and medical departments. His experiences in these aggressively non-philosophical settings persuaded him to write practical philosophy books for health professionals. The real world continues to drive his writing, even after nine books for Wiley in twelve years.

David moved to Auckland in 1992 and is now a citizen of both Britain and New Zealand. He lives happily alongside the Tamaki estuary, with his wife Hilary and daughter Charlotte, and for some reason enjoys a consistently warm welcome from Ed, the local bottle-shop owner.

# Preface

If you are a health worker and you want to understand ethics you have two choices. You can study texts which take ethical principles for granted, or you can read books inspired by a theory of health. Both types discuss practical cases, but with a profound difference.

If you plump for 'principles first' books you step into quicksand. Different texts espouse conflicting axioms. Read enough and you'll find ethical principles behind every practice. Pro- and anti-abortion lobbies both have ethics on their side. There's a school of thought that considers health care rationing morally abhorrent, and another that thinks efficient resource allocation is what ethics is all about. Some societies claim that health services are morally special, others believe they sell commodities like any other business.

How do you choose between contrasting moral allegiances? And how do you respond to colleagues who do not hold your ethical beliefs? If they are utilitarian while you feel duty-bound to offer everyone equal care, how do you argue with them? If they insist they are right you'll never change their minds just by telling them they aren't.

You can escape the stalemate if you have a theory of health. If you do, your reasoning need not start with blind moral faith but with careful deliberation about the *point* of working for health in practical situations.

If you share the philosophy of health that informs *Ethics: The Heart of Health Care* then your moral outlook is not a purely intellectual matter either. If you choose to uphold this philosophy you make a commitment born of centuries of compassionate practice. And once you've made it you no longer have to barter principles. It is pointless to protest – 'this practice is unethical'. However, a practically relevant justification is essential:

> 'Excuse me doctor/nurse/manager/policy-maker, but what are you trying to achieve here? What is the purpose of your intervention? What inspires your behaviour?'

If you get an answer you can debate fundamentals – not ethical whims. What notion of health does the response suggest? What would happen if the idea were applied consistently to all health work? Where does this understanding of health goals differ from your own? *Is* yours better? Why?

Because work for health is a moral endeavour it must be thoughtful. And because careful thinking matters so much it is not acceptable that health care decision-makers hide behind status, codes of practice, ethical biases dressed up as truths, or even the law. Whenever you ask – *how does what you are doing create better health?* – nothing less than honest, reasoned answers will do. This book will help you get them.

DS

# Preface to the First Edition

This book extends a theory about the nature of health into the heart of practice. It is genuinely philosophy applied. And it is long overdue.

In the majority of areas of human activity there exist theories, sometimes a range of competing theories, about the meaning of a particular activity, about its limits, about the sorts of methods and techniques that are most suited to it, about its implications for other areas of activity, and about the moral issues that are raised by it. Such theories are usually known as philosophies. So not only are there specific human activities known as medicine and social science, for instance, but there are also branches of inquiry which try to analyse and understand the rationale of the practices.

Thus there is a philosophy of medicine and a philosophy of social science which aim at uncovering the *raison d'être* of each discipline. Since the philosophies are concerned with the underlying reasons for the practical activities so they inevitably have an influence on the future development of them.

Work within the philosophy of medicine may ask, for instance, whether treatments in medicine should be given *at any cost*, or whether there are occasions on which it is better not to treat patients. The philosophy of social science asks questions about what forms of inquiry are truly to count as social science, and about how much faith can be placed in the reliability of any results generated from inquiry in social science. The answers offered in response to such theoretical questions can have immense practical impact on the parent activities.

It is, at first sight, puzzling that there is no discipline concerned with the philosophy of health. Given that health work periodically affects every member of society (at least in the Western world) from a time before birth until death it is surprising that so little attention has been given to its philosophy. A partial explanation for this phenomenon is that 'health work' is a term with such a wide variety of meanings and applications – from open-heart surgery to political action over environmental hazards – that it is extremely difficult to identify it as a single coherent body of activity. Also, many of the constituent parts of health work – such as medicine and social science – already have their own philosophies.

However, it has been shown[1] that health work can be delineated – albeit within a broad boundary – and that this process of delineation and clarification can have implications for practice. For instance, some forms of practice – say, drug trials carried out on patients without their knowledge – can be seen to be work for health in only a very limited sense, if at all. And other practices not normally considered to be work for health – say, talking to a person to help him picture his social circumstances in a more realistic way – can now be seen to be work for health in a very strong sense. Clarification can change the priorities of practice.

*Ethics: The Heart of Health Care* further pioneers the exploration of the philosophy of health. By charting the extent to which moral issues permeate work for health, by demonstrating tangibly and graphically that *work for health is truly a moral endeavour*, a solid and useful theoretical basis for health workers of all kinds is created. From this platform health workers can grasp more firmly the theoretical significance of their everyday activities. Having gained a stronger grasp on theory health workers are placed in a far better position to appreciate the extent to which they have a huge personal responsibility for the health care they give. Such responsibility is frequently demanding and trying, but if it is handled with confidence it can also be exciting and fulfilling.

# THE ARGUMENT OF THE BOOK – PHILOSOPHY APPLIED

It is time that philosophy is again recognised for what it is. Philosophy is an essential part of the way in which we understand our world. It is a process of inquiry that can have real practical effect. The best philosophers are not happy merely to 'watch the wheels turn'. They know that what they do can help produce better wheels, or even rearrange those wheels so that a different machine is created. Philosophy can rejuvenate practice.

This book makes the following points and connections. It forms a powerful guide for those in health care who wish to work with a high degree of morality, and who would also like to improve the structure and organisation of health care.

- The world of health care is undergoing a period of intellectual crisis, quite separate from the current political and economic debates on the funding and cost-effectiveness of the NHS. There are a number of forces that are challenging existing assumptions and patterns of practice. These forces include rising interest in holistic medicine; increasing pressure by lay people to have access to medical secrets, including their own medical records; pressure to include the study of medical ethics in undergraduate curricula; and the arguments of some social scientists and health promoters that work for health must begin in society rather than focus on individuals.
- The tension between old and new ideas can be illustrated by an idea borrowed from the philosophy of science – the notion of 'paradigm shift'. It is best to think of this notion only as an analogy rather than a reality. The old paradigm – the old set of cherished beliefs and principles – is being called into question by the new forces. Hence a period of crisis exists in which conflicting ideas and principles do metaphorical battle.

   The process of change from one paradigm to another is not definite and predictable. The future must, to an extent, be shaped actively by people. The question is: *How is it possible to ensure that the new era of health care that emerges from the period of crisis has the best possible form and content?*

- The route to an answer is opened up by offering health workers a more comprehensive understanding of the nature of ethics. Ethics is the key to the new era of health care. Health workers must know that *work for health is a moral endeavour*.
- But work for health is not a moral endeavour in the sense of a crusade. It is not a moral endeavour in an evangelical sense. The task is not to identify what is good and bad, right and wrong, as a dogmatist might. Ethics is not a discipline in which pure blacks and whites can be uncovered and then applied for ever without further question. Ethics is always a question of degree, a question of deliberating about which interventions in other people's lives will produce the highest possible degree of morality.
- But how can the degree of morality of an intervention be assessed in any objective sense? Both ethics and health work are beset by the problem that people in complex societies have different values and beliefs. What one person believes to be a good intervention in the life of another, an intervention exhibiting a high degree of morality, another person might regard as a poor intervention. Even advice about diet and exercise is never based wholly on fact. At some stage a value judgement of some kind will be made.

  The extent of the influence of value judgement can be seen from the ten case studies [15 in the second edition] presented in Chapter Four. There are no clear-cut solutions to any of the situations presented, and whatever solution is proposed must involve some reference to values. Since people's values frequently conflict, how, if at all, can a firm theoretical basis for consistent moral intervention be given to which all health workers can assent?
- There is a range of answers which fail.

  1. One might search for the 'objectively good'. In other words one might pursue some ultimate value or ordering of values which is truly moral. But there can be no means of uncovering the 'truly moral' since in ethics much depends upon personal opinion and subjective judgement. It is not possible to discover the 'objectively good' as one might discover Mount Everest, or a solution to a problem in applied mathematics.
  2. Alternatively, one might search for a set of rules, or a code of practice, to provide a firm uncontroversial basis. However, experience shows that whatever rule, or set of rules, is selected there are always exceptions. There will always be courses of action which offend the rules but lead to the creation of a higher degree of morality than if the rules had been obeyed.
  3. One might appeal to law, but a similar problem to that of the appeal to rules arises.
  4. Or one might instead settle for a relativist position, where it is accepted that there is no objective standard of morality, where what is to be done depends upon judgements made at the time under the existing circumstances. The trouble with this option is that morality can become a meaningless term. Given sufficient advocacy any form of intervention might become permissible for a time. Current law might prohibit some actions, but the higher court of appeal – the court of morality – will be left powerless.

- Where is the foundation for consistent moral intervention to be found? An appeal has to be made to the facts about human nature and potential. Although it is very hard to determine what a truly good human potential or action is, it is less difficult to establish which actions are truly bad. It can be shown that certain ways of limiting human beings – ways of *dwarfing* people mentally, physically, and spiritually – are plainly immoral. Consequently, moves to prevent *dwarfing*, examples of attempts to liberate the enhancing potentials that people possess, form a basis for the most moral health work.

- How can this assertion be given support? Attention has to be paid to the definition of 'personhood'. What is a person, and what forms of human potential, out of all the possibilities, are the most important and significant? The view is advanced that the mental life of a person, which forms an essential part of the definition of 'personhood', is at least as important a target for health work as a person's physical life.

- It is important that health workers are in a position to apply the results of this analysis. So, with relevant and accessible examples, traditional theories of moral philosophy are explained. Too often in the past these theories have been left to languish in a scholarly vacuum.

- However, even with this theoretical background and firm base, there remains much uncertainty and room for conflicts of values within the ethics of health. But this is simply the nature of ethics. *The* right course of action cannot be prescribed as if it were a pill for a specific ill. There will always be legitimate alternative courses of action that might be chosen.

- Because of this constant need for deliberation and balancing of principles, a tool – the *Ethical Grid* – is offered to health workers both as an illustration of the nature of moral reasoning and as an aid to choosing actions to produce the highest degree of morality. Through the use of this tool health workers have the means to justify their choices, to explain how these choices might be shown to be the most strongly opposed to *dwarfing*.

  The Ethical Grid is not a calculating machine. It is merely a euphemism for 'ethical reflection'. It can produce different solutions to the same situation dependent upon who is using it (that is to say, dependent upon who is deliberating). But it does enable health workers to be clear about what is immoral by indicating the range of interventions which lie beyond the limits of the grid. And by giving a clear core rationale the grid allows health workers a basis on which to decide for themselves between alternative possible interventions.

- Finally, recalling the ideas of crisis, paradigm change, and ethics as a key, some implications for the future of health care are considered. Principles such as 'respect for autonomy' and 'respect people as equals' have become likely new priorities for health work. If these principles, and others contained within the core of the grid, are accepted by those with the power to alter the shape of health care, then it will take on a different form. One possible new structure amongst many alternatives is sketched out to show how philosophical investigation – the process of clarification coupled with proposals generated out of logical analysis – can carry true practical weight.

Here, at last, are the beginnings of a philosophy of health.

Green Park
London, UK
September 1987

# Acknowledgements

## ACKNOWLEDGEMENTS TO THE FIRST EDITION

During the period in which this book was created my life took on a life of its own. This was a strange and crazy life which refused to tell me what it intended to do next, or why. Fortunately this other life never found out about the book. I deeply thank Alan Cribb and Annmarie Carlen for helping me keep the secret.

Both these friends were of immense practical help, as were Harry Lesser and Mary Brown. The Departments of Community Health and General Practice at Liverpool University kindly allowed me the necessary time to write the book, and the Health Education Authority allowed me the necessary money to pay my bills.

There were various other influences on my life which must also be acknowledged. My other life would like to thank Ulrig and Martha from Metz for introducing it to a novel sport, Gabby from Florence for introducing it to the Italian version of Teutonic efficiency, and Luxembourg for not being any bigger. There are also thanks due to Chrissie Adams (Zandra Rhodes under a cobalt sky with Standards), my lawyer, Chorlton Water Park, the Nitromors Co., and an ever-circling squabble of dingoes for continuing to circle. Further gratitude is due to 16 December 1986, 20 February, 28 April and 26 September 1987, and to Frank and the boys for not designing the cover to this book. There will always be a special place in the heart of my other life for Duffy Seedhouse. Although this boy is now ten years old he has never once uttered a word of complaint or protest.

## ACKNOWLEDGEMENTS TO THE SECOND EDITION

My other life left home shortly after the first edition was published, and I haven't seen it since. As for Duffy, he's as quiet as ever, the dingoes have been rounded up and shot by Australian conservationists and Frank has a job designing CD sleeves for AC/DC. *This* life would like to thank 25 May 1991, 26 September 1992 and – especially – 23 June 1996.

# Introduction

There ought to be two reasons why this book has been successful but I suspect there is only one. *Ethics: The Heart of Health Care* has been studied for a decade because it offers down-to-earth guidance to those who want to analyse ethical problems for themselves.

Its practical elements were devised partly to meet a personal need. Between 1984 and 1987 (when the book was completed) I was a junior researcher in a department of health studies, and later a lecturer in a post shared between departments of general practice and community health. My degrees were in philosophy, and I had a reputation for asking apparently facetious questions: What is health? What is special about your work as a nurse? What are the limits of your professional role, doctor? Why I was employed in these institutions was not – I confess – immediately obvious to all my colleagues. However, interest in ethics was escalating in the mid-eighties' health world (for reasons I did not then properly comprehend) and I became known as the local 'ethics person'.

## TEACHING ETHICS

I quickly learnt that in academic institutions burgeoning interest in a subject does not necessarily imply a similar level of resource with which to study it – in fact there is sometimes a strikingly inverse relationship between these factors. There was usually no room for ethics in official curricula, and the meetings I was asked to lead were squeezed into lunchtime slots or stitched into other courses (they still are sometimes). All of which meant that I typically had no more than 50 minutes to explain ethics from scratch to groups of strangers.

My earliest attempts suffered not only from lack of time, but from my ignorance of the practicalities of orthodox health care. A novice of health service reality teaching newcomers to ethics over a snatched sandwich was unlikely to be an overwhelming success. I would try to explain different theories in moral philosophy while my students would patiently introduce me to such essentials as medical/nursing hierarchies, 'not for resuscitation' notes, and the irrationality of health service decision-making. On the best days both parties would each learn a little from the other, but we never managed to get beyond the basics, and were rarely able to begin analysis proper.

Despite these repeated stumbles, it became clear both that I would continue to receive invitations to teach ethics to groups of health workers, and that I was unlikely to be allowed more time to do it. I needed something more if I was to continue to accept these offers – I needed a framework which would enable me to present complex ideas rapidly and accessibly, and which would also ensure that realistic solutions could be offered to the students' endless practical problems.

This was asking a lot, but I did have assets on which to build. I had already developed a theory about the importance and purpose of health work, I had a brilliant friend and colleague to talk to, I was willing to make a compromise between the purity of philosophy and the murkiness of practice, and I very much wanted to be useful. These attributes combined to produce the Ethical Grid.

## SPIDER'S WEB OR ETHICAL TEMPLATE?

If I had not been able to discuss health care ethics and how to teach it with Alan Cribb I would not have come up with the Ethical Grid. I remember a conversation with Alan over a beer (several in my case) in a Manchester pub. We were discussing the pervasiveness of ethics in health care, and bemoaning the perception that ethics is only of peripheral concern for health workers. I think I may have asked Alan to tell me the main components of health ethics, as he saw them.

I cannot recall the details, but I was struck by the image he proposed. He said – I think – that it is an error to think of key or organising principles in ethics. Rather one should conceive of ethics as a 'spider's web' in which each idea is connected to all other ideas by all manner of routes, and where each is partly responsible for the strength of the web as a whole. In different circumstances different parts of the web may be more useful than others, but all may be needed – a fly can land on any part of a spider's web, after all.

But Alan's idea was not that ethics is a way to 'trap a problem'. He was explaining that wherever one starts in a deliberation (whether one considers rights, duties, consequences, virtues or principles) if the deliberation is done thoroughly one will either have to visit the other areas at some point, or will receive implicit support from them. If you are a doctor anxious to know whether you have a duty to tell your patient's partner something she wants kept secret, you must reflect on matters beyond duty (What will happen if I do this rather than that? Who will benefit? Who will suffer? Who is entitled to know what? Is negotiation possible? Is there a way to avoid confrontation?). Good ethics is comprehensive deliberation about the pros and cons of action.

Alan had expressed a powerful insight into the nature of ethics, and I thought for a while that this might be the answer to my teaching problem. However, what was enlightening to me – a trained philosopher – proved too complicated for the inexperienced audience I was trying to teach: I needed something equally philosophically illuminating, but simpler to apply.

Somehow the 'ethical web' changed, in my imagination, into a much less beautiful piece of engineering. I pushed, pulled and chopped it until it became a group of simple, transparent squares, on each of which a key ethical word or notion was inscribed. My idea was that this 'ethical template' (as I then saw it) could be 'placed over' a situation by the reasoner and – dependent upon which part of the template was superimposed – could bring a solution into focus.

This was not a good idea, not least because it was too rigid – the antithesis of the understanding of ethics Alan and I shared. For example, I had in mind something like the sketch in Figure 1.

However, the association of boxes was not only arbitrary but also fixed. Most problems would require boxes from various parts of the template – a box from here, another from there – so making superimposition impossible.

My next proposal – almost as inadequate as the static template – was to design the teaching tool to resemble a game in which the player moves squares in a fixed frame. One square is missing and the challenge is to juggle squares round this space until the required arrangement is produced (in some versions of the commercial game the aim is to arrange numbers or letters in the right order). I envisaged the ethical reasoner moving transparent pieces until he hit on the right combination to 'place over' the ethical problem, as shown in Figure 2.

Not only was this too cumbersome, it also had the effect of focusing the reasoner's attention more on the 'game' and how to move the squares around than on the ethical problem itself. I had to find a way to include all the essential squares and words within a clearly defined structure (to help students grasp immediately that ethical analysis can be kept within bounds), but with flexibility of use and interpretation.

The next attempt, Figure 3, looked too much like a dartboard. So in the version published in the first edition I retained the idea of angular movable boxes but removed them from the over-restrictive frame. Instead I arranged them in four distinct layers

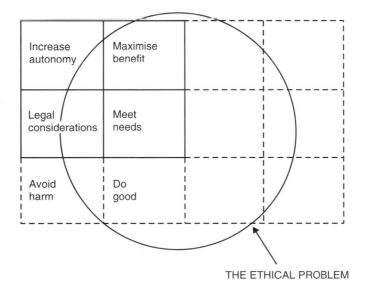

**Figure 1**   The ethical template superimposed over an ethical problem

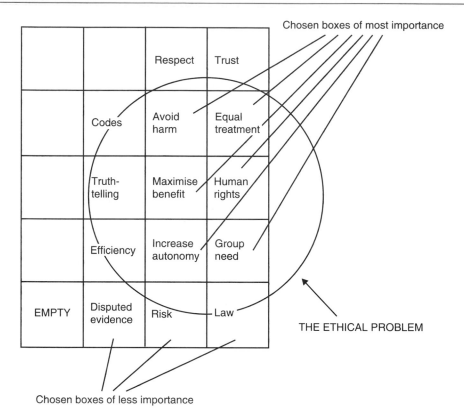

**Figure 2**    Movable boxes in the ethical template

(see p. 209): black for practicalities, green for outcomes, red for duties and blue for health work purpose. This gave the Grid sufficient rigidity to prevent disorientation amongst new users while permitting considerable fluidity of application (though the Grid is not infinitely malleable (see p. 208).

## THE SECRET REASON FOR THE BOOK'S SUCCESS

If this had been all there was to my thinking, if *Ethics: The Heart of Health Care* was merely the Ethical Grid plus summaries of ethical theory, and the Grid little more than a loose collection of coloured labels, I would not have published. If I had intended the book to be 'gimmicky' or 'ethics by rote' as some unperceptive reviewers seemed to think, I would have been wasting my time writing it. Worse, I would have been deceiving readers about the nature of health care ethics, when my real purpose was to facilitate improved deliberation about pressing practical problems.

Because the book is so accessible and uncomplicated I fear that both general reader and scholarly critic alike have tended to overlook just *why* it is so clear. The book looks so straightforward it is hard to imagine there is more to it than meets the eye. But there

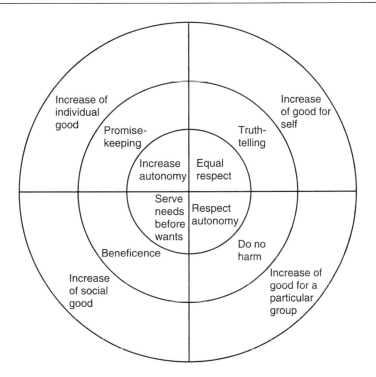

**Figure 3** Part of an experimental circular version of the Ethical Grid (Early 1986)

is. It is not written in an elaborate 'academic style' – non-academics can understand it – and it is simple in the most positive sense of the word. But it is also theoretically rich. If it were not underpinned by a strong theory it would not be so easy to read, and I have no doubt it would have suffered the fate of countless more scholarly ethics books, consigned to one small print run and then isolation on some obscure library shelf.

In this Introduction permit me the luxury of outlining the hidden reason for the book's success. Let me explain first that *Ethics: The Heart of Health Care* is Part II of a still growing series – the sequel to an earlier book and one part of a now sizeable body of work. Allow me to add a little more theory – let me explain the moral importance of *committing* to a theory of health. Let me briefly summarise what some may have missed in the first edition. And finally let me tell a frightening personal story which renewed my ethical fervour, and brought home just how much further there is to go.

## Foundations Two

In 1985, two years before I wrote *Ethics: The Heart of Health Care*, I completed the manuscript for my first book, *Health: The Foundations for Achievement*.[1] This project sought to discover a theoretically and practically defensible answer to the question: what is health? Various theories of health were surveyed and discussed, and each was found wanting in important respects. However, my analysis revealed that all theories of health (certainly all the theories I came across) and all practical work done in health's name, stated or implied that work for health is done in order to remove actual or perceived obstacles to the achievement of biological or chosen human potentials. Health work, in other words, aims to liberate fulfilling human potential by the prevention, elimination or alleviation of impediment: the nurse offering a careful explanation to an excitable patient, the general practitioner sending blood samples to a lab for testing, the psychiatrist seeking the best combination of medications to reduce a patient's mental turmoil, the public health specialist investigating the cause of an outbreak of food poisoning – each of these is doing what is professionally expected and each is working to tackle obstacles to desirable and/or biologically normal human growth.

In *Foundations* I developed this observation into a theory of health intended to display the theoretical limits to health work, and so help practitioners work out more exactly what their role is – to help them decide when they should begin to intervene, which interventions are legitimate and which not, and when they must withdraw from situations. As I developed this theory I was at the same time developing an account of the ethics of health work, though I did not realise it at the time.

*Health: The Foundations for Achievement* does not mention ethics. Though it may be hard to believe, I was so taken up with conceptual analysis I was oblivious to the work's ethical content. I wanted to find out the meaning of health and to show that knowing this could improve practice. It was only later, as I taught my work to a nursing class and gave ethics sessions to other groups, that I slowly put two and two together. I came to understand that there is not one compartment labelled 'the theory of health' and another labelled 'health care ethics', but that it is impossible to think deeply about health without also thinking deeply about morality – and vice versa.

Most books on health, medical and nursing ethics do not appreciate this connection. Instead, their authors take commonly held ethical principles and apply them to health care contexts.[2,3,4] They have not been developed with health care in mind, and can be applied equally to other social situations. It is rare to find much theoretical support for these principles, and even more unusual to come across reasons why these and not other principles should be brought to bear on health care situations. Unlike *Ethics: The Heart of Health Care* these books tack ethics on to health care. This book, by contrast, is rooted in an understanding of the nature of health (taken from *Foundations*) and develops its ethical argument (and the Ethical Grid) out of this.

The slogan 'work for health is a moral endeavour' is not a throwaway line but meant to announce that there are striking commonalities between what it means to work for health and what it means to be engaged in practical moral deliberation. 'Work for health' is a morally special activity, its purposes more humane and noble than most other human enterprises (including commercial activity, the system of adversarial criminal law, and pure mathematics, to give just three examples).

Note too that 'work for health' does not mean only traditional health care, such as doctoring and nursing. These activities can be work for health but are not necessarily so. The terms 'health care' and 'health service' are sometimes used in this text to mean 'medical care' and 'medical service', but it should be remembered that this is not an automatic conjunction. If medical services are not carried out in line with the foundations theory of health then they are not health work (in the *Foundations* sense).

## WORK FOR HEALTH REQUIRES MORAL COMMITMENT

It may be helpful to expand on this point. The body of the book argues that there are no moral standards beyond the human world (or the world of persons, more technically). This means that no one is morally obliged to act in any particular way – if you want to behave selfishly no 'moral court' will ever punish you. However, since all social behaviours take place in the moral realm, we continually have a golden opportunity to commit to moral ways of life – if we choose. Those who genuinely wish to work for health must make a knowing commitment to achieving health goals – and this requires commitment to a theory of health. As she commits, the health worker pledges simultaneously to a powerful set of moral obligations – a commitment all the more emphatic because it is voluntary.

If ethics means anything then:

i. Actions, made by competent human beings, which have relevance for other human beings, inescapably have ethical content because they have the potential to affect others for better or worse

and

ii. All competent human beings have the capacity to recognise this.

## ETHICAL A AND ETHICAL B

(i) and (ii) form part of a theory in which there are two forms of the ethical, *ethical A* and *ethical B*, where *ethical A* means *ethical in the sense of having ethical content* and *ethical B* means *ethical in the sense of having a consistent view about what one ought to do in the social world.*

*Ethical A* is a pervasive phenomenon of (competent) human life. Because we live with others in an ethical realm we constantly encounter ethical situations, whether or not we perceive them as such. Being pleasant, unpleasant (or anything else) to people during a Saturday morning trip around the supermarket are *ethical A* actions – regardless of intent – because they have the potential to produce different sorts of meaningful consequence.

Not every action is *ethical A*. Those of no relevance to other people lie outside the ethical realm. Idly playing with one's hair, tapping on the desk as one works, reflex responses such as the blink of an eye and so on, are not of ethical interest. Only if they become potentially or actually relevant to others are they *ethical A* actions (if desk-tapping is done in a shared office or if hair twirling becomes an obsession which could interfere with one's relationships, for instance).

*Ethical B* actions stem from a person's awareness that what she does is socially important. The task for anyone who wishes to be *ethical B* is first to work out what 'being ethical' means, and then to devise the most effective strategy to be it. Since the founding question of ethics is *how should I conduct my life in the presence of other lives*? the ethical challenge – at any time and in any place – is to work out what *commitment to living* to make. When a desk-tapper who wants to be ethical realises she is being irritating, it is up to her to work out what to do about it. She might decide to stop – or she might reason that she is entitled to continue – but whatever she decides, as she sees that her actions have implications for other people and resolves because of this to behave in a certain way, so she begins to create her *ethics B*.

## Health Work Ethics

Work for health is a certain sort of moral endeavour – a certain sort of *ethical B*. Not only is it generally true that actions made in the social world by competent human beings inevitably have ethical content, but health work – probably more than any other work – *exposes* this *ethical A*. Even something habitually dismissed as trivial – a smile for instance – is more obviously within the ethical realm in medical work than it is in most other fields of human endeavour: a condescending smile offered to a sensitive and vulnerable patient might be extremely damaging, while a sincere smile of welcome could emancipate. Furthermore, because the *ethical A* is so visible in health work, most health workers find it necessary to commit to some *ethics B* or other. Normally these *ethics Bs* are either vague (forms of everyday ethics – see p. 37) or based on principles and beliefs derived from sources outside health work (as is the case with almost all positions in medical ethics). Yet it is immeasurably preferable that health workers practise according to a properly thought out theory about what health work is and why they ought to do it.

Health workers should take as much *command* as they can of the *ethical A* by committing to an *ethics B* based on the foundations theory of work for health. The Ethical Grid is a graphic illustration of this. Its three outer layers are analogous to the *ethical A*, and the blue layer is a simple summary of the *ethics B* I recommend to health workers. It is this *ethics B* that is meant to govern the Ethical Grid.

In Figure 4 the iceberg represents the ethical realm. The matchstick person must live as part of this realm, whether he likes it or not. He must also, if he wishes to *be* ethical, make a commitment to an *ethics B* – to a particular way of living in the social world. To do this properly he needs help. He needs a method to enable him to see the full extent of the iceberg (*ethical A*), and to structure his thinking as he seeks to achieve ethical goals consistently. If he wishes to be a health worker he must commit to an *ethics B* based on a theory of health. He will achieve all these ends if he makes good use of the Ethical Grid.

## THE BOOK'S ARGUMENT

The particular argument of *Ethics: The Heart of Health Care* also seems to have gone largely unnoticed. It is not clear why (its main steps are spelt out in the unaltered Preface to the first edition). It is worth restating those points that have been most misunderstood, in the hope the book might yet be seen for what it was meant to be.

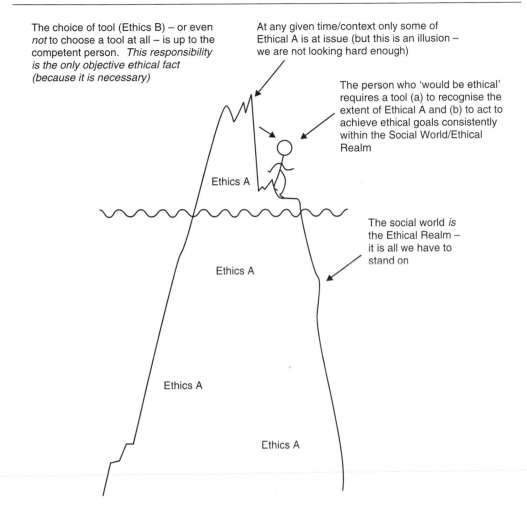

The choice of tool (Ethics B) – or even *not* to choose a tool at all – is up to the competent person. *This responsibility is the only objective ethical fact (because it is necessary)*

At any given time/context only some of Ethical A is at issue (but this is an illusion – we are not looking hard enough)

The person who 'would be ethical' requires a tool (a) to recognise the extent of Ethical A and (b) to act to achieve ethical goals consistently within the Social World/Ethical Realm

Ethics A

The social world *is* the Ethical Realm – it is all we have to stand on

Ethics A

Ethics A

Ethics A

**Figure 4** Ethical A and Ethical B illustrated by use of the iceberg

A cursory look at Chapter One may give the impression that my case was not only naïve, but entirely wrong. It may seem that I was merely (and falsely) predicting an imminent paradigm shift – wagering that a version of health care based on my theory of health would shortly supersede health care based on no theory of health. A more careful reading of Chapter One will show I was hedging my bets, but I concede that I was hoping that health systems would have moved closer to my ideal, ten years on. I even expected it in optimistic moments. Yet if anything health systems have become less like Paradigm Y than ever.

Although I did not realise it in 1986–88 (as a young philosopher I was still insulated from the practical world by my training, even though I had begun to work in a health environment) much more influential landmarks were being put in place in the UK, where I was living. I had thought – with woefully little evidence – that the rather romantic list I give on pp. 4–5 of the first edition amounted to a signpost showing health care's near-future direction. And in this I was wrong, and had missed the writing on the wall in front of me.

Not only had US academics and policy-makers been debating the escalating costs of medical care in that country for two decades, but the Conservative government in the UK was increasingly taking notice of what they had to say. The Tories were rightly concerned that the British NHS, largely run by medics and administrators, was set to absorb ever greater amounts of GDP unless something was done to control spending. Their answer, following a review in 1983, was to introduce 'health management', informed by commercial notions and supported by advice from economists (soon to be commonly known as health economists). In ensuing years this has meant greater emphasis on 'value for money', demonstrable 'outputs', quantification, and squeezing as much as possible out of increasingly demoralised staff. Indeed it looks as if Paradigm X has been replaced not by Paradigm Y but by Paradigm Z. It looks as if the old guard, who think health work should be guided by medical priorities, has been overrun by an army of managers who are not particularly concerned what drives the system, so long as its costs are kept in check.

My speculations about the content of Paradigm Y were admittedly idealistic and ill-informed – but then they were meant only as speculations, nothing more. I hoped things were going to get better quickly, but I was to be disappointed. However, speculation aside, I was attempting to offer a solid argument.

1. The crisis that really concerned me was not that which still worries UK and US governments. I was not bothered about transient policy matters. I was interested in the *conceptual* crisis I had discovered as I was researching *Foundations*. I was concerned about the fundamental health care problem, which was that no one – as far as I could tell – was clear about the point of it. No one could properly define the purpose of health care, and without this health workers were bound to remain vulnerable to political whim and policy fad.
2. It can be shown that medical services are not necessarily synonymous with health services. Because:

   > A person's or group's (optimum) state of health is equivalent to the state of the set of conditions which fulfil or enable a person or group to work to fulfil their realistic chosen and biological potentials[5]

   not only can work for health be done without reference to medicine and medical priorities but medicine can be practised without it being work for health.
3. Many health workers were dimly aware of points 1 and 2 but found themselves frustrated, powerless to do anything to change things for the better. Not only could they not specify what 'better' meant in practice, but they did not possess sufficient theoretical grounding to move toward it.
4. I hoped to offer disaffected health workers the theoretical backing they needed. Since work for health is a moral endeavour it was obvious – to me at least – that if I could help health workers learn how to reason morally (by drawing on a thoughtful combination of moral theory and health philosophy) then their daily practice would provide the impetus for the new era to come, sometime in the future. That is:

   > The theories people hold about their everyday work – the subjective theoretical framework in which they operate – can affect their interpretation of what they do. Health

workers' understanding of their practice affects both their performance and their attitude towards those for whom they are caring. Since a variety of subjective understandings exist it is surely important to make them overt . . . By so doing . . . it may then also be possible to shape future developments to correspond with the richest sense of health, by highlighting the most moral understandings of the point of health work . . . it may just be possible to speed the formation of Paradigm Y, to ensure that it emerges with the most enlightened and egalitarian rationale (see p. 30).

Similarly:

The process of change from one paradigm to another is not definite and predictable. The future must, to an extent, be shaped actively by people. The question is: How is it possible to ensure that the new era of health care that emerges from the period of crisis has the best possible form and content? The route to an answer is opened up by offering health workers a more comprehensive understanding of the nature of ethics. Ethics is the key to the new era of health care. Health workers must know that work for health is a moral endeavour (see p. xiv).

5. The Ethical Grid is meant to enable health workers to inject Paradigm Y theory into their everyday practice.

It is impossible to show that answers to practical problems are absolutely ethical. However, it is clear that the deliberate and avoidable *dwarfing* of persons (i.e. most human beings – see Chapter Six) is fundamentally immoral, and that the further health workers can distance their practices from dwarfing the more moral their work will be. Some answers are more ethical than others because they liberate more and better potentials.

The Ethical Grid combines moral theory, health theory and pragmatic context. In addition, the requirement that reasoners use at least one blue box is meant to ensure that practical solutions are inspired by the foundations theory.

The fact that ethical deliberation can produce varying and even incompatible solutions does not undermine the speculation that by doing ethics a better shaped health system will emerge. Rather, it is the act of reasoning, critically, honestly and where possible publicly, that will bring about the revolution.

At present too much health care (which is still popularly taken to mean the provision of medical services) is organised hierarchically, and too many health workers are not allowed to think for themselves. Protest is stifled, tradition holds sway, people are able to get away with crass judgements just because they have senior posts or are medically trained, and resources are allocated not through the force of reason but because certain individuals have greater power than others. Of course this is the way of the world. Corruption is part of human life, but there are degrees of it – it is possible to have more or less corruption, to have a more or less principled system, to be more or less honest, and to work according to specified theories or not. Things do not have to be the way they are and I maintain, despite the surface evidence, that progress can and will come once enough health workers genuinely and consistently practise ethically, in the sense put forward in this revised text.

It is idealism to imagine that a device such as the Ethical Grid could become a ubiquitous tool of practice – it is too unsettling, too levelling, too challenging to the status quo – but I have seen it used to good effect in enough different situations (in critical care, in paediatrics, in nursing, in oncology, in neonatal units) to know that it can work and that health workers feel greater confidence when they use it. Indeed, through using the Grid and studying *Ethics: The Heart of Health Care* thousands of practitioners have discovered that intelligent moral reasoning requires neither formal philosophical training, nor the blind acceptance of dogma. It is not unrealistic to hope that its use will become more widespread still. Perhaps – just perhaps – sufficient health workers will take advantage of it to bring about a tangible shift in the ethos of health care.

# THE OPERATION

I was recently vividly reminded why it is so important that Paradigm Y materialises.

I have been developing my position for over thirteen years, and had become lulled into thinking that everyone was aware of it. Of course this was a feeble assumption, but nevertheless an easy one to make. Worse still is to assume that not only does everyone now see your point, but they are also acting on it.

The extent to which this is a false belief hit home recently, during an unwanted encounter with an Ear, Nose and Throat surgeon. I relate the tale to show how easily – and how much – harm can be done in ethical ignorance.

## A PERSONAL EXPERIENCE

For as long as I can recall I had a small, firm, roundish, mobile lump below and slightly forward of my left ear. I didn't worry about it, just fiddled with it occasionally as I shaved (it seemed insignificant and stayed the same size). I mostly forgot it completely. Sometime before Christmas 1996 I noticed it again. It seemed a little bigger, but I couldn't be sure. In any case I couldn't imagine it would be serious. I'm healthy and expect to stay that way, after all.

In early December I went to the GP for a couple of things and mentioned it to her. I could tell, from her immediate distraction, that it might be serious. Instantly I began to feel sick (sick to the stomach and sick that I was in trouble and sickest that this might affect Hilary – my wife – and Charlotte – my daughter). The GP, who seems to have an intuitive understanding of the relationship between ethics and work for health, was straight and to the point:

'You'll need to see an ENT surgeon. You may need an operation. Do you have medical insurance? No? Well it may cost $2000–3000 so we'll try the public system first.'

I stuttered some questions, mostly to establish just how much I should worry.

'I'm 99.9% certain that it isn't cancer. I know what a cancer feels like. I used to work in a hospice.'

'Should I worry about this?'

'No.'

But I did, of course. Dazedly, with the help of Hilary's characteristically perceptive prompting, I wondered. If it's nothing to worry about why do I need to see the ENT surgeon? What exactly is this problem? And later that evening, if it is going to cost $3000 then what will the operation involve?

I managed to put the problem to the back of my mind for at least some of the time and got on as best I could. Just before a brief holiday in Nelson I received an outpatient appointment to Auckland hospital, which made trepidation unavoidable.

I went to the hospital *worried and ignorant*. I emphasise this because – though I'm probably over-anxious – I imagine the great majority of patients in similar situations must feel as I did. And I emphasise it because it must surely be obvious to anyone seeing people in such circumstances that this is how they must be feeling.

After a wait of three-quarters of an hour, in a crowded waiting room, unable to establish how long I would have to wait despite politely asking the receptionist, I was shown into the consulting room by a nurse. Will I get my lump cut out here and now? I thought. I hoped so. I hoped it would be a local anaesthetic and that would be that, but I was forlorn to see a small room, not surgically equipped. I knew already that my worrying would have to go on.

The doctor wasn't there and the nurse was trying to be cheerful – I can't remember what she said but she seemed more nervous than I. She scurried around like a giant mouse. She was about to rush away with my notes when I managed to ask if I could see them. 'Of course', she said, 'these days you have a right to', but she was in so much of a hurry I could read no more than the GP's referral letter which asked for the surgeon's opinion on excision, with the brief history I had given. Thoughtfully my GP had highlighted in pink the sentence: **the patient is senior lecturer in medical ethics at the medical school**.

The surgeon, a conspicuously overweight middle-aged man, breezed in. I stood up – I think he may have held out his hand to introduce himself. He immediately said 'where's this lump then?' and felt it as he wished. Almost instantly, or so it seemed to me, he announced 'you have a benign tumour of the salivary gland' (I didn't know if I was relieved or shocked – I certainly had no idea what this meant). He then directed me toward the examining table and told me to lie down. 'I just want to take a needle biopsy' (I think this was what he said). He didn't ask for permission, and he didn't say there might be any untoward consequences (other than the obvious one of finding out that I had cancer), and I was obedient. It all happened so quickly it is hard to see how I could have objected without causing considerable fuss.

He took his needle and inserted it into my lump. 'This might hurt a bit.' 'Yes' I said. What else do you say? It did hurt a bit – not much, though it hurt more when he wiggled the needle around inside the lump.

As he was doing this he was speaking. Something along these lines:

'So you're a lecturer in ethics are you? Where?'

'At the medical school, across the road.'

'I've not seen you before.'

'I don't see many surgeons.' (This was an attempt at a joke. It went unnoticed.)

'I don't bother with the medical school any more – too socialist for me.'

'Oh no', I said, looking at the nurse out of my left eye, between the needle and the surgeon's arms. She raised her eyebrows. In sympathy, I think.

He squirted the sample between two microscope slides. As he did so he called his registrar in.

'This is Dr blah blah.'

'Hello', I said.

'This patient has blah blah blah.'

What did he say? Before I had time to ask, registrar blah blah had said, 'That's all I need to know' and left the room.

'Thanks, Doc.' I managed.

I was told to sit up and to return to the Dr's desk. I felt shakier than ever.

'You need an operation but there is a risk.'

'OK' I said. 'What!!?' I thought. He showed me what needed to be done. He reached under his left ear and with his right hand made as if to pull back a large flap of skin, just as a cartoon character would remove a mask.

'It is not easy to get at the blah blah. There is a less than 1% chance of damage to the facial nerve. Even if all goes well you'll have a sore left ear and your ear lobe will almost certainly always be numb.'

I couldn't believe this. This wasn't happening.

'What's the worst that can happen?' I was convinced he was going to say 'you'll die'. But he said nothing. Instead he took his finger and pulled the left side of his mouth firmly downwards.

'Oh God' I thought. I knew I wasn't right but I hadn't expected this.

After I told him I hadn't got insurance he put me on the waiting list for the public hospital .

'How long will I wait for?'

'I can't say, you know what a mess the public system is in at the moment – it could be months.'

'Does that matter?'

'No, but the tumour needs to be removed.'

Without meaning to, he then reassured me.

'I won't ask you to wait for the result of the biopsy because I'm virtually certain what it is.'

'When will I know for sure?'

'If you don't hear within a week it is what I think it is.'

At some point – whether before or after this I can't recall – he said, 'Of course, if you went private it could be done much quicker – I have a private practice but I'm not supposed to tell you that here.'

'How much?'

'It could be four and a half thousand.'

'You'd better give me your card.'

'I don't have a card here, but here is the number of my private rooms.'

There were several questions floating in my mind – and I wasn't so thrown I'd forgotten what they were – but he was pointedly waiting to leave so I only managed to put a couple – and these had to be prompts to him.

'So, if I don't have this removed it gets bigger and then that can cause damage?'

'Yes.'

'You think I should get this done?'

'Yes.'

And that was that. I gave my form to the receptionist and reeled out of the ward, unable to think straight, with months of anxiety ahead. I went to my office across the street and called Hilary. She was shocked and upset but had the presence of mind to advise me to call my friend, a retired physician. I told him I had a benign tumour (I hoped) of the salivary gland, and it was from him I learned it was technically a tumour of the parotid gland (though that wasn't what the doctor had said to the registrar, I was sure).

Because I work in a medical school I have access to the library so I read up what I could. I wasn't sure what sort of tumour I had (I discovered there are different sorts of benign parotid tumour) but my friend – on further inquiry – told me he thought it was most likely a mixed-cell tumour. And if so it should come out because though they grow slowly they don't stop – one book had a picture of a man with one the size of a football – and they can suddenly become malignant (which was worse news than ever, but I was so emotionally deadened by now it didn't matter very much).

I told Hilary and we decided to pay for the operation out of our savings. I called the surgeon at his private rooms. After a couple of hours he called back (to his credit he didn't then know that I wanted a private operation). I told him I'd decided to pay and asked when he could do it.

'I'm going on holiday soon but I could do you on Tuesday if you like.' It was Thursday at 4 p.m.

'OK' I said, my thoughts muffled in a nightmare.

I pulled out of it, and discovered more about parotid tumours from an Internet site. This helped explain the doctor's reasoning (my symptoms fitted a pattern typical of a benign tumour). Two days later I had cause to read the site more carefully still.

## A Cricket Test

On the Saturday, aware I was overanxious about what might happen, I took myself off to the New Zealand vs England cricket Test at Eden Park, Auckland. But though the sunshine baked me I felt bleak, and couldn't concentrate. For no particular reason I decided to move to a seat in the West Stand. As I walked behind the South Stand to get there I was shattered – utterly shattered – to realise that my mouth had filled with blood. I spat it out, oblivious of the spectacle I might make to the other people milling around, but the blood kept coming. Swallowing most of it I went to the Gents for water. I swilled my mouth and saw in the mirror that the lining of my cheek – behind the tumour – seemed to have irregular lines of blood leaking from it.

I felt as if I wasn't there. That's it, I thought. I've had it now. It's cancer and I'm going to die. And at that point I again had the feeling it didn't matter. My – presumably irrational – reaction was if that's it that's it and there's nothing I can do now.

But the blood stopped. It went as quickly as it came. White-faced I bought a diet coke (I had been intending to do this anyway) and walked as if weightless to the West Stand, where I sat in disbelief. No more blood though.

I couldn't sit at the cricket – so I drove to work (a mile away) to phone Hilary. I didn't want to but had to tell her what had happened and we were both upset. I was on the verge of tears, but the bleeding had stopped so I rallied.

I called the doctor's mobile phone but it was switched off. I called his rooms (no answer – it was Saturday). I called the hospital – maybe Dr blah blah the registrar can tell me what it is. I got through to him and explained what had happened. He was quite unconcerned. I think this was actually disinterest but I interpreted it favourably and – as I had done with the surgeon – prompted an answer which had only just occurred to me.

'I assume – I hope – that the blood is something to do with the needle biopsy?'

'Yes', he said casually, 'there are many small ducts which lead to the inside of the mouth. The surgeon must have damaged some, and they must then have clotted. The clot dissolved, that's all. It's nothing to worry about.'

'It's nothing to worry about if you know what it is' I said, with surprising force considering my mental state. But he didn't rise to the bait and said – once I told him I had opted for the private operation –

'I'm sure you'll be all right once my boss has operated. As my grandfather used to say, "a stitch in time saves nine".'

Good grief, I couldn't help thinking, he'll be telling me a spoonful of frigging sugar helps the medicine go down next, but I left it. Thanks Doc, I said to him for the second time.

I checked on the Internet site. Sure enough, here were the risks of needle biopsy, none of which the doctor told me before he took the sample. They are:

Advantages

- – Safe, economical, easy to perform, minimal pain.
- – Often provides a preoperative diagnosis and may obviate the need for surgery in some patients.

Potential Problems

- – Haemorrhage.
- – Fistula formation.
- – Facial nerve injury.
- – Infection.
- – Needle tract implantation.
- – Interpretation difficulties.[6]

Thanks Doc, I thought.

## AT THE HOSPITAL

The ethically barren pattern continued at the hospital, and I confess I found it difficult to cope. It is important to appreciate how I was feeling – a doctor's moral incompetence always has a human context.

I didn't sleep much the night before my operation, partly because I had to be at the hospital by 7 a.m., and I never sleep well if I know I have to wake before five. But I got through the night and cycled (yes, cycled) the fourteen or so kilometres to the Medical School.

The morning was dark and warm. I had a tail wind and hardly a car went by. Despite my fears it was impossible not to feel some comfort in the subtropical tranquillity that cradled me.

As I walked to the hospital – a private one twenty minutes away – I began to be upset. I was plain scared of what was to come – the pain, the risk and the unconsciousness. But more than this I despaired at my powerlessness – I had opted to place myself in a situation where I knew nothing and could do nothing. I found this paradox impossibly frustrating but still I walked toward it, forcing tears away.

I arrived and sat in the foyer waiting to be admitted, observing three other equally miserable new patients with sympathy – and horror that I was one too.

I was shown to my room by an auxiliary. What I saw drove home further (as if I needed it) that despite the floral bedsheets, neat TV and new carpet, I was not booking into a hotel. They were going to cut me soon and I would be on this bed later, bleeding and hurting.

On the wall by the bed was a bag containing plastic tubes for breathing, a panel of switches with an 'emergency aid' button, and a bag holding a LIFE AID℠ resuscitator. Standard issue daily apparatus, trivial to a doctor or a nurse, but its presence paralysed me. How can I be here? They don't have resuscitators in hotels. There is nothing I can do now. It was agonising to lose independence so quickly and casually.

A nurse, Charleen, checked me in perfunctorily. I must have sounded scared but she was either unwilling or unable to offer me the reassurances I needed, despite my asking her as many open questions as I could think of: 'Is he a good surgeon?', 'What sort of anaesthetic will it be?' (I wanted her to say 'Oh, a 100% safe one, you'll love it'), 'How many ops does he do at this hospital?' As we were completing the consent forms the surgeon entered. I stood up and made as if to shake hands, a gesture he either did not recognise or chose to ignore. 'Have you still got the lump?' he asked, presumably in jest. 'You know I have', I replied half in annoyance and half-bemused. He then took out his purple marker, drew a ring around the lump and started to leave.

'Is that it?' I spluttered incredulously.

He stopped. He was slowed anyway by the tight squeeze between Charleen and the wall of my room. Charleen also looked at him, unintentionally forcing him to take a step back toward me. I moved back too, so I could face him squarely.

I can't remember if he said anything. I think he probably didn't. But I know I managed to say – straight out and again with a courage that surprised me, 'What about the biopsy? What was the result of the biopsy?' I can't recall the exact words but he indicated, brusquely, that it was OK.

'So it was a pleomorphic adenoma?' I offered.

'Yes.'

'So I don't have cancer?'

'No.'

'Well that's something good at least.'

And at that he left, with a flabby wave and a 'catch you later'.

———————— ◆ ————————

It may be that this was an exceptional experience. But there was every reason for the surgeon to behave all the better with me since he knows I lecture in ethics. Furthermore, according to the nurses he is by no means 'the worst'. So I assume it is not exceptional. Indeed there is evidence all around that it is not – Paradigm Y has yet to take shape – and this is not good enough.

What, I would like to know, did the surgeon think he was doing? What was he trying to achieve? I hazard that he did not know what he was doing because (a) he had no goal other than to do his surgery well (which he did and for which I am thankful), (b) he had no moral plan, (c) he had no moral reasoning skills, and (d) (worst of all) he is unaware that he has a daily theoretical, intellectual and practical challenge equally as demanding as his surgical function – though of a different kind.

I do not deny that what matters in the long term is that he did good surgery, but this is not to say that his short-term failure is therefore unimportant. For all we knew it could have been as long term as it was going to get. I could have died and my final five days would – in some part due to his moral negligence – have been amongst the most wretched of my life. And even though it turned out that these days were a small episode in my history, they did matter. They were important to me and my family, and they could have been happier had my doctor properly grasped what it is to work for someone's health.

And what is most shocking about this depressing state of affairs is that it is so *obviously* unacceptable. I have made this point before, I make it elsewhere in this second edition, and no doubt I will continue to make it for years to come: the medical profession does not properly understand its role. Most doctors (and many other health professionals too) think clinical work is an end in itself – that medical activity defines its own purposes – but they are wrong.

My anaesthetist did a good job, as far as I know, and I felt no serious pain during or after the operation (though the surgeon was right about the lasting effects). This is as it should be and no doubt my surgeon was happy about this – anything less would have been unacceptable. Clearly one of the main aims of the operation was to avoid pain, to make sure that I was not disabled by this obstacle to my potential.

If the anaesthetist had failed to control my pain when it was within his power to do so then he would not have achieved a central goal of his work. Equally, and I insist on *equally* at this point, if any health worker in any respect within his capabilities fails to control a person's pain in general when it is in his power to do so, he will have failed to achieve a fundamental goal. People suffer mental pain too.

It matters profoundly that health workers act comprehensively. This is why I wrote this book in the first place, and why it is worth presenting it afresh, in the hope it will give new impetus to Paradigm Y.

## THE NEW EDITION

It is ten years since I wrote *Ethics: The Heart of Health Care*, and much has changed in the meantime. If I could start from scratch today's book would scarcely resemble the original. Rewriting it has reminded me just how raw the first edition was. When I wrote it I was young – not yet thirty when I began – excited and in a hurry. I had invented the Ethical Grid and I wanted the world to see it. I did not want to publish it in an academic journal my intended audience would never read – I wanted it in an accessible book with case studies, exercises and explanations about ethics.

I was so keen to get it out that I rushed the writing. I usually write countless drafts until I get the meaning and rhythm just so, but this book took only two. I knew I was going too fast, but it hardly seemed to matter. I thought I was a better writer than I was, but mostly it was a heady experience and I was carried away by it.

I have tried to compromise in this edition. The writing is less ambiguous, I have refined some points in the light of later work, and I have cut down the repetition. In the first edition I was aiming to guide readers step by step through the book, so I included summaries and reminders at regular intervals and more than once made the same point in different places. This is not always a bad thing, and I have retained some reinforcements. I have also added two further decision-making aids, adopted from *Liberating Medicine*, a text-book written three years after *Ethics*.

The first edition was an honest, innocent exploration, and I have done my best to retain this freshness. When I began the project I did not have answers to the questions: What is ethics? What is the relationship between health and morality? and How can philosophy help health workers with practical decision-making? I found out as I wrote. I hoped to convey this sense of quest to the reader, so I presented the book as a search – a hunt for the moral, to paraphrase the original title of Part Two. I wanted the reader to share in the exploration – to wonder where it would lead and to attempt her own answers as she went along. It is only by engaging with philosophical problems that philosophy is learnt, so I wanted my questions to bother the reader too. I wanted them to become her problem – so she might work out her own ways forward, and could fully appreciate the Ethical Grid at the finish. I still do.

David Seedhouse
Auckland, New Zealand
September 1997

# PART ONE

# Work for Health is a Moral Endeavour

# CHAPTER ONE

# Growing Pains

## IN THE MIDST OF CRISIS

The health world is so conceptually disoriented it sometimes seems it may never achieve its moral potential. Mostly we bumble along – perpetually troubled by territorial squabbles and inadequate resources – blind to the intellectual challenge that must be met if health work is to become all it can be.

Despite repeated practical success, health care lacks a coherent account of its purpose.[5] All notions of health (and so of what health care is meant to accomplish) stem from social values. Not everyone favours the same set of values, so different accounts of health care purpose co-exist. But which of them is the true version? Which form of health work is most ethically justifiable? Which interpretation of health ought to guide health policy? How can we reach a philosophically secure decision about the aims of health care? Few members of the health world appreciate the full significance of these questions, and fewer still offer sustained responses to them.

The conceptual crisis has not appeared overnight. Nor will it be resolved quickly, though there have been important developments during the past three decades. The British health service, for instance, is more open to non-medical innovation than it has ever been,[7] and medical schools are increasingly keen to offer students a wider and more intellectually demanding education.[8]

These and other forces are challenging the traditional view that medicine has an exclusive right to define the nature of health care. But there is no deliberate rebellion. For the most part the crisis is coming to a head spontaneously, as health care evolves and matures. It is becoming increasingly apparent to thoughtful observers that questions about what health systems are meant to achieve, and how ethical reflection and medical practice are related, must be comprehensively answered. Despite the fact that they are not often officially heard, and despite recent unimaginative stop-gap 'reforms',[9] the dawning conclusions to these questions have massive implications for the provision of health care.[10]

## LANDMARKS (1988)

Landmarks stand out in this health care revolution. Among the most prominent are:

- Rise in the popularity of alternative methods of treating disease and illness, several of which clash with traditional medical theories of disease.[11]
- Growing interest in holism and holistic medicine.[12]
- Acknowledgement by some clinicians that medicine must reassess the nature and causes of disease, and realistically contemplate the extent to which medical interventions are effective.[13,14]
- Recognition, in medical education and beyond, of the importance of ensuring meaningful communication between doctors and patients. Many medical schools now emphasise how important it is that doctors genuinely understand patients' worries. Modern schools teach that doctors should be warm, approachable and empathic, should be able to engage in clear dialogue and – where appropriate – be capable of encouraging and helping patients to cope with their problems themselves. Of course, correct diagnosis and appropriate prescribing are as important as ever, but this shift is fundamental nonetheless – it is an expansion of the traditional medical understanding of the point of health care, and it has wide ramifications.[15]
- Increasing awareness in the medical profession that the role of clinicians in health promotion is – at least potentially – less significant than that of politicians and environmentalists.[16]
- Impetus to include training and examinations in ethics for medical under-graduates.[17–19]
- Pressure from nurses to drag nursing courses away from the old idea of training in technique toward the additional goal of providing students with higher education in an academic setting. Nurse education must still produce skilled and competent nurses, however the 'new nurse' is a thoughtful carer armed with sufficient knowledge and experience to form her own judgements at work.[20]

## LANDMARKS (1998)

The above landmarks remain – indeed each has become more obviously pivotal since 1988. But change is slow. The health world's inability to embrace a philosophy of health means that some events which looked like landmarks in 1988 were of little significance, and some were altogether false.

In 1988 the medical establishment appeared more flexible than it actually was. Nurses have not been widely accepted as independent practitioners; there has – with the advent of the health manager – been some change in health service hierarchies, but if anything this has tended to narrow the focus of conventional health care;[21] health promotion has lost its way, baffled by a blizzard of rhetoric and naïve idealism;[5] and moves to offer health care in the community – too often inspired by the desire to save money – have met with mixed results.[22] Academics – especially those in secure, tenured employment – might have been expected to lead the way: to dissect, explain and propose theoretically sound improvements to the often blatant irrationalities of the present systems. But too many are spineless – they find it much more profitable to go along with the status quo.

# AN IMAGE IS CHANGING

Nevertheless, the idea that it is desirable to provide health care solely according to clinical priorities (ignoring social and moral aspirations) is now under pressure. Medicine has dominated orthodox health care because of its high social status and hefty financial muscle, and because its practitioners have privileged knowledge. But although these features are constant, and health work appears as controlled by medicine as it ever was, beneath the surface inspirational conceptual developments are taking shape, even though the majority of health workers are still not aware of them.

## THOMAS KUHN'S THEORY OF PARADIGMS

Thomas Kuhn's theory of paradigm change[23] is a handy way to illustrate this, though it is not claimed (in this book) that paradigms really exist. Kuhn's work offers a helpful shorthand image of a complex process, but it is not clear what a paradigm is. The version offered below is one of several possible accounts.

Kuhn, a philosopher and historian of science, was interested in the history of scientific research. He investigated the attitudes and beliefs of research scientists and found that for most of the time – usually for their entire careers – most scientists have common aims, accept the same standards and procedures, and embrace shared criteria of success. They engage in what he calls 'normal science', where they try to solve 'puzzles' – or technical difficulties – within an accepted tradition. Occasionally, however, scientists are faced with a crisis which causes them to question the most basic assumptions of their research tradition. When this happens what was thought to be bedrock can turn to quicksand, and everything may be thrown into uncertainty.

Typically, during a paradigm change events and results of experiments are observed for which the current set of explanations (the paradigm) is unable to account, a phenomenon accompanied by a growing perception that the existing way of seeing things is inadequate. This perception, that 'there is something profoundly wrong about the theoretical framework in which we are working', can develop into an intellectual crisis which – after often rancorous debate, and a sometimes desperate search for a more satisfactory direction – may be resolved only by redefining the entire project. Such redefinition is possible only when the most politically powerful researchers have become convinced it must be done.

## A CLASSIC EXAMPLE OF PARADIGM SHIFT

The change in perspective when Newton's theory of mechanics was superseded by modern physics is often cited as a classic example of a paradigm shift or scientific revolution. Newton's theoretical structure was applied fruitfully for over two centuries.[24] However, as developments in technology both demanded and facilitated increasingly precise measurements and predictions, Newtonian mechanics was found not quite accurate enough. It was discovered to be impossible to increase accuracy further within the tradition. Instead Newton's mechanics was supplanted by another theory, one which explained the evidence in a radically different way. This was not a steady progression but a dramatic upheaval – a remarkable revolution in thinking. The implication of this for our understanding of the nature of science is immense since it calls into question the 'common-sense' that science is a steadily accumulating body of public knowledge about reality.

After studying similar historical examples it seemed to Kuhn that 'common-sense' is mistaken, and that spectacular changes in direction can and do take place within well-established research disciplines, even those that have achieved considerable practical success. Newton's stature as a scientist and original thinker is unshakable, yet modern physicists no longer build on his physical theories. Good research can be done which produces fundamentally mistaken hypotheses, so progress in science cannot only be a matter of adding to existing work. Sometimes accepted theories and wisdoms have to be reassessed and rejected. Furthermore, this process can happen in all research traditions, not just in natural science.

Many philosophers disagree with Kuhn, arguing that it is both arbitrary and melodramatic to call a series of explicable developments a 'revolution'. Some critics point out that if the history of science is studied with care there are always strands of continuity to be found.[25] However, while Kuhn's theory of paradigm change clearly does not provide a complete explanation of the growth of scientific thought, it is nevertheless enlightening to explore his idea in relation to contemporary health care. To do so is inevitably to oversimplify, but it can help show how the idea of paradigm change might encourage a more complete appreciation of health care change.

## THE HEART OF THE CRISIS IN HEALTH CARE

A 'paradigm shift' looks like Figure 5, where Paradigm X represents the old consensus, and Y its successor. The overlap symbolises the common ground remaining. So far as the classic example is concerned, Newton and his contemporaries can be thought of as working in Paradigm X. When it was discovered that Newtonian mechanics could not explain some astronomical observations this paradigm was thrown into crisis and a new one eventually assumed dominance. In physics Paradigm Y, which was to give birth to Relativity theory, the uncertainty principle, and quantum mechanics,[26] was a radical departure from Paradigm X. Many of its basic assumptions contradicted Newtonian theory, although some beliefs were still shared. For instance, the use of logic and mathematics, the demand that all theories should be tested as rigorously as possible, and the terminology of the old paradigm, remained common.[25] In other words, even when a radical shift occurs the two spheres are not totally separate. Some philosophers of science maintain that the shift is neither as neat nor as simple as the Venn diagram illustration suggests, and that it usually makes more sense to think of the new paradigm as encompassing the old one, retaining the 'falsified knowledge' and mistaken beliefs, but finding this information of little or no relevance to future work (see Figure 6).

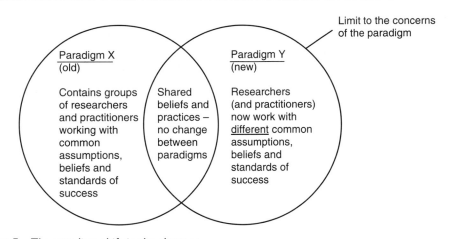

**Figure 5** The paradigm shift in the abstract

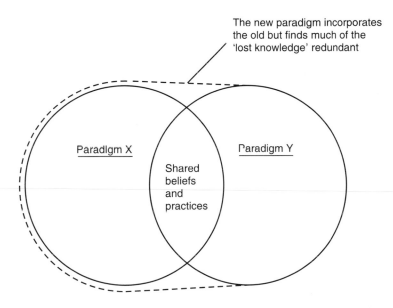

**Figure 6** The new paradigm encompassing the old one

## RELEVANCE TO HEALTH CARE

The notion of paradigm change may be employed in the world of health care as an aid to understanding. However, even this very general idea is not wholly appropriate, since health care is more to do with practice than research, and Kuhn's interest lay mostly with scientific theorising. Nevertheless there is a partial analogy. For instance, the present situation might be thought of like this (a caricature included merely to illustrate the idea of paradigm change).

## PARADIGM X

Paradigm X contains the 'old school' of health care where health is thought to be nothing more than the state of a person not suffering from disease, illness, or infirmity; where the medical profession defines its rationale without consulting those whom it seeks to serve; where the idea of medical education is that as many facts as possible should be crammed by students (who soon come to see their 'education' instrumentally – something to be got through to become a doctor); where the idea of providing students, who daily will have to make crucial decisions about the lives of other human beings, with a proper grounding in ethics is seen as pointless – or worse, seen as a threat; where technical decisions are made 'for the good of the patients' without patients' involvement; where patients are used to test the effect of drug treatments in controlled experiments without their knowledge; where patients are not permitted to see their medical records; where the health service is organised in strict hierarchical lines in which everyone knows his or her place; where curing disease through clinical science is the primary motivation; and where measures of success or failure in the care of patients are predominantly quantifiable, emphasising severity of disease, degree of deviation from statistical norms, and life expectancy.

## PARADIGM Y

Paradigm Y is the fruition of the developments and initiatives listed on pp. 23–24, plus other practical improvements. It is based on a different theoretical understanding of work for health – its impetus is the simple idea that people are of fundamental consequence. In Paradigm Y curing disease and illness and increasing the length of life remain important, but are not always as important as increasing the autonomy of those who request or need health care, distributing available resources fairly, education, and respecting people's choices even if they conflict with given advice (although there are limits to how far the choices ought to be respected – see Chapter Ten).

Paradigm Y policy-makers understand that health in the richest sense can be more to do with personal freedom than physical fitness. Its health services are organised to ensure all workers have a say in what happens to it; the users of the service are allowed to see whatever has been written about them and, as far as circumstances permit, are involved in all decisions that affect them. The task of enabling people to develop mentally, physically, and emotionally – creatively throughout their lives – is a primary motivation (see Figure 7), necessitating a restructuring of most services.

Paradigm Y has not yet crystallised. The rudimentary version just outlined is a suggestion only, but it is by no means out of the question today.

## A HIDDEN CRISIS?

Many in the health world still do not think Kuhn's image has anything to do with health care, and will dismiss the initial premise of this book. Any evidence of a health care 'crisis' is at best superficial, they will say. The conventional position is that there have

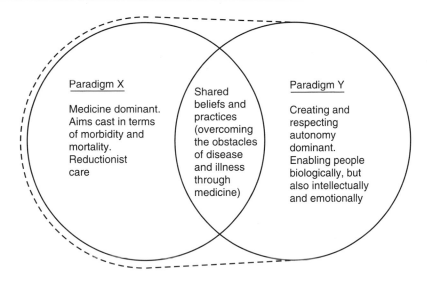

**Figure 7**   A possible paradigm shift for/in health care

been some changes of emphasis (this is in the nature of human endeavour, after all), and some secondary developments (such as holistic medicine) which complement the main body of medical work. But slow evolution hardly constitutes intellectual crisis, and clinical medicine rightly governs health work.

These critics might be right – Paradigm Y may turn out to be a hopeless dream. However, it is worth remembering that during his investigation into the history of scientific research Kuhn noticed that during the 'crisis period' – the time when two paradigms are competing for ascendancy – only very few people recognise that a transition is taking place. Some may suspect a revolution, but it is only with hindsight that the true extent of the crisis becomes apparent.

It would not be too surprising if so much foment were to escape the attention of busy health workers absorbed in particular tasks. There is little enough time to reflect on changes even within our own disciplines. Standing back to take a view of health care as a whole can appear impossible to those daily involved in dealing with the many distressing obstacles that hinder patients. As with political revolutions, for all of us working during the transition, it may only be when the dust has settled that we will see the complete picture.

## THE GESTALT-SWITCH

Kuhn uses a further illustration to back his claim. He argues that the change of perception that happens when an individual notices he is working in a new paradigm can be likened to a 'gestalt-switch', an idea derived from the Gestalt school of psychology which flourished at the start of the twentieth century. The school criticised the Behaviourist account of perception, which held that complex sensory events were nothing more than the sum of individual nervous impulses. The Gestalt school argued that some perceptual experiences show that a person's own contribution to what is seen cannot be ignored if a full explanation is to be given, and that sometimes the whole (the Gestalt) experience is more than the sum of sensory impulses. As one example, they explained that the presentation of several photographs, each only slightly different from the one before, in rapid succession to give cinematographic motion, is not actually motion. Members of the school pointed out that all the eye has received is a number of discrete still photographs, yet the subjective perception is of movement. The only possible conclusion, they argued, is that the brain adds to the sensations it receives – so human beings have a unique part to play in the creation of the realities we experience.[27]

The gestalt-switch idea is famously illustrated by showing that an arrangement of lines on paper can be seen in different ways. The pictures in Figure 8 might be either a duck or a rabbit, and either a vase or two faces, according to what we think we are seeing. There are two points to note here: that the theories we have about what we are observing help us make sense of what we observe, and that it is necessary to have a relevant theory in order to make sense of anything. Kuhn's insight was to extrapolate this idea into the realm of science where if we hold one theory (say Newtonian mechanics) we 'see' the evidence in one way, yet if we hold an alternative theory (say the new theory of physics) we 'see' precisely the same evidence in a different way.

It is perhaps not over-stretching the point to develop this line of thought in a way germane to the future of health care. The theories people hold about their everyday work – the subjective theoretical framework in which they operate – can affect their interpretation of what they do. Health workers' understanding of their practice affects both their performance and their attitude towards those for whom they are caring. Since a variety of subjective understandings exist it is surely important to make them overt – to reveal them to their holders as they really are. In this way health workers will see that beliefs they take to be self-evident are not obvious at all (they will see there is a range of plausible alternatives) and it may then also be possible to shape future developments to correspond with the richest sense of health, by highlighting the most moral understandings of the point of health work. In this way it may just be possible to speed the formation of Paradigm Y, to ensure it emerges with the most enlightened and egalitarian rationale.

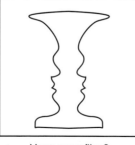

Vase or profiles?

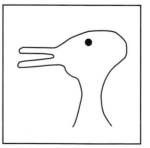

A duck or a rabbit?

**Figure 8**   Examples of the gestalt-switch

# HEALTH WORKERS CAN CREATE FUTURE CHANGE THROUGH PRESENT PRACTICE

The degree to which paradigms are determined is an open question. Perhaps events unfold according to some blueprint, perhaps human beings have no say at all in what happens to us. However, speculations about the extent to which we have free will, or are merely pawns in some celestial game, are intriguing but must remain inconclusive.[28]

Given this uncertainty it is wise to assume that human initiatives can affect the future, at least to some extent, and prudent to believe that the shape of the new paradigm is partly up to health workers. The paradigm is bound to change sooner or later. It is up to health workers to ensure that the best features – those features truly part of health work in its fullest sense – finally crystallise.

What health workers do now – in everyday practice – will be instrumental in bringing about the future of health care. We are constantly faced with choices which will shape our destiny.

Our paths are limited by what we have done, by our talents, our education, our circumstances, and the historical era in which we live, but we almost always have some choice about what to do, what to believe, how to act towards others, and what to say. Even in circumstances where our choices are restricted, alternatives are usually open to us. For instance, a teacher may have no choice but to teach a class of disinterested and unruly teenagers, but still have significant options about how best to deal with them. And even where choice appears totally limited we can at least choose between doing and not doing a thing. We can create ourselves, more than we think. And just as we can create ourselves, through our actions we can create conditions in which *other* people are better placed to create more fulfilled versions of themselves too.

During the paradigm transition, it is vital that health workers not only *speak* of 'positive health' and 'empowering' but also *act* according to richer ideas of health. A person's actions are the acid test of his beliefs. It is, for instance, not good enough to believe that individual autonomy should be a priority for health work – and should sometimes be placed above the duty merely to prolong life – and yet to conform in practice to the latter principle. If the best new paradigm is to triumph over the failing one, then health workers who believe in it must ensure they are true to themselves, and that their actions match their opinions.

# DISEASE OR HEALTH?

The gestalt-switch analogy can also help explain the central tension at the heart of the paradigm shift. Gestalt-switch difficulties can be overcome, and the way to do it is to display and explain both options simultaneously. This is not so difficult. Do you want to see either a duck or a rabbit, or do you want to be able to say, 'I see them both. Now I can make up my mind which I prefer'?

## Clarification of Meaning is Crucial

The nature of practical work for health is reciprocally related to health's meaning, so clarification of meaning can make a difference to what is done. If work for health is only taken to mean work to cure disease then the implications for practice are substantially different from those which follow if work for health is taken to mean 'liberating all human potential to the fullest degree'. In an earlier book,[1] various meanings and theories of health were discussed, among them the views that 'health is a state of complete physical, social and mental well-being, not merely the absence of disease, illness and infirmity', the theory that health occurs when disease is absent, the theory that a person is healthy if she can perform her normal social function, and the theory that health is a strength – an ability to cope with or adapt to the problems life throws in people's paths. These theories are not fully compatible with each other. They will not gel into a coherent whole without contradiction. For example, a person might have a disease (and so be unhealthy according to one possible meaning of health) and yet still be able to perform her normal social function (and so be healthy according to an alternative meaning of health).

The analysis offered in *Health: The Foundations for Achievement* reveals a common theme beneath the various theories. This is that work for health is always designed to remove obstacles in the path of biological, intellectual, emotional, and creative human potentials. The *Foundations* argument is that health is a richer idea than commonly supposed – health is to do with human flourishing, not merely the absence of disease. Effort against disease can be genuine health work, but it is not the whole story.

The *Foundations* analysis can make it easier to see the health world's gestalt-trap – the noose in the middle of the crisis. Consider the hypothetical job title 'Health Promotion and Disease Prevention Officer'. This label is not implausible, and would certainly make sense to many health promotion advocates.[5] The fact that two separate terms – 'health promotion' and 'disease prevention' – can be used together implies different meanings. By reflecting on these it is possible to highlight a tension, as yet only faintly perceived by many, between the idea that health is dynamically yet inextricably linked to disease alone, and the emerging view that health is truly to do with the extent to which a person is equipped to live a fulfilling life.

Much of the ambiguity in health studies has come about because this major distinction seems invisible. Forward-looking authors writing about health frequently introduce nebulous ideas like 'positive health' and 'well-being' to indicate that health is not one side of a seesaw counterbalanced by disease and illness. But then, having glimpsed one picture momentarily – having seen a duck and not a rabbit – even the most radical health promotion visionaries slip back into the old habit of discussing how to decrease disease and illness.

Health writers and workers caught in the trap fleetingly realise that health is to do with fulfilment, but then they hit a daunting mental block. As soon as they begin to consider how this fulfilment can be made concrete, they fall back under the spell of medicine, hurtled backwards as if attached to a piece of elastic stretched as far as it can go.

The problem is that health is still habitually thought of from a point of reference which begins with disease, and this is such a powerful idea that almost everyone seems to think that if talking about health one must necessarily refer to disease, illness, handicap and injury sooner or later – or else you cannot be talking about health at all.

Health educators and promoters provide a clear example of the gestalt trauma (or at least the example is clear once one can see both sides of it). Many health educators continually insist that health is more than the absence of disease and illness, yet their official work is almost entirely directed at preventing disease and illness. Having experienced a fleeting insight into the fullest sense of health the very next thought of the ensnared health educator is always something like, 'How can I persuade this person to adopt the kind of habits which will make him less prone to becoming ill?' Certainly, if a health educator can achieve this particular goal then she stands a good chance of enhancing a person's life in general (for instance, if the person who is the target of the persuasion avoids a stroke as a result then this will prevent a wide range of obstacle, not just brain damage). The trouble is that constant emphasis on ameliorating disease and illness in the name of health embalms a central mistake – the continuation of the unreflective assumption that preventive and curative medicine is the best means of helping an adult person to become more of what she could be. Yet of course it is not. Health is not only a matter for medicine and can be created and improved in numerous ways for which medicine has no brief.

## SUMMARY

So far it has been suggested that:

1. A range of forces symptomatic of an intellectual crisis in the world of health care can be identified.
2. The idea of paradigm change has been introduced in an elementary way, in an attempt to illustrate the nature of the crisis. Whether or not paradigms exist is immaterial. Health workers need only acknowledge that change for the better is possible.
3. It is in the nature of human affairs that a new pattern of health care will eventually crystallise. It is to be hoped that this new framework will be based on ideas drawn from a richer view of health than is currently popular.
4. Although forces can be identified which seem to compel the paradigm shift it is impossible to predict its nature. The future of health care is not predetermined.
5. It falls to health workers to ensure that the best alternative becomes reality. A great deal hinges on how health workers think and act.

## THE NEXT CHALLENGE

The tasks for health workers are these:

1. To understand that a range of ideas about the purpose of health care exist.
2. To expose the ideas which inform the richest possible work for health.
3. To act according to these ideas as soon and as often as possible.

And so

4. To ensure that the new paradigm is the best possible theoretical framework.

But how is all this to be done? How can such a mammoth task be attempted coherently? How can a set of principles be agreed upon by people with divergent interests? How can the ambition to create a new era of health work be achieved without being destroyed at birth by political dispute? How can the principles of the new paradigm be explained so that they assume their true significance, above the pervasive pragmatism of administration, staffing, resource allocation, and battles over mini-kingdoms?

## AN ANSWER

The answer is at once stunningly simple and frustratingly complex. It lies in the fact that there is a fundamental link between the idea of health and the idea of morality. This link has not, even now, been noticed to anything like its fullest extent.

Health work is moral work. Consequently, by making clear the range and importance of the moral content of health work, by bringing what already exists to the fore in its proper focus, it should be possible to bring about the most desirable form of the new paradigm. Ethics is the key to the formation of health work's new era.

# CHAPTER TWO

# Ethics is the Key

Most people regard ethics as at best a secondary concern in health and medical work, and some (health economists, for instance)[29] believe ethical issues are not relevant at all. But they could not be more mistaken.

It will become clear, as this inquiry develops, that far from ethics being of peripheral interest, it is the key which can release thoughtful health workers from their gestalt limbo. Ethics stands at the very heart of health care, and can unlock the exit from the crisis. Creating health requires ethical commitment. Work for health is a moral endeavour: this is the catchphrase of the new paradigm.

## WORK FOR HEALTH IS A MORAL ENDEAVOUR

The slogan 'work for health is a moral endeavour' should not be used without understanding the reasoning which lies behind it. But once the supporting arguments are known, the expression can serve as a constant reminder of the reasons why working for health is so important – and is an invaluable starting point when explaining the connection to others who do not yet realise how good the future of health care could be.

### A Possible Objection

But what does the slogan mean? How, it might be asked, is work for health a moral endeavour? Health is undoubtedly desirable – but a person's state of health is not a moral matter. People either are or are not healthy. Being moral is not to do with how people are – it is to do with what people do. Ethics starts and ends in exceptionally difficult situations in which judgements must be made about what is morally right. Given this, surely it is a confusion to mistake being healthy for being good?

### A Response

It is not claimed that a healthy person is a good person, nor is it asserted that health workers should be crusaders for some particular moral creed. Rather it is argued that work for health in its richest sense is equivalent to acting morally, in a thoughtful, purposive fashion.

This relationship is not easy to grasp since it involves many further definitions and distinctions that are explained later in the book. However, it is immediately necessary to understand that moral questions are very rarely cut and dried. It is better to think of morality as a matter of degree – ranged on a continuum running from the immoral to the highest degree of morality – where the precise nature of the various degrees, and their rankings, is mostly an open question.

To associate the ideas of morality and health in the way described in the above query is a fundamental mistake. The moral element of health work does not come into play only when specific dilemmas arise. Ethics is not only to do with such sensational questions as 'Should we switch this life support machine off?' or 'Is it right for a doctor to prescribe contraceptives to a fifteen-year-old girl against the wishes of her parents?' or 'Should all seriously intellectually disabled women be sterilised?' In fact ethics permeates all aspects of health work. Morality is of such profound importance in health care that it is impossible to understand the nature of health work without also understanding the nature and purpose of ethical reflection.

# WHAT IS ETHICS?

## INTRODUCTORY REMARKS: ETHICS IS COMPLICATED

(Note: in this book no distinction is made between 'ethics' and 'morality'. All variations of each word may be used interchangeably.)

Because ethical reflection is meant to give answers to questions about how men and women should act, the scope of ethical concern is immense and varied. This diversity can be dissected into different types, the analysis of which can become involved (as any survey of texts in moral philosophy will show) since most contain a range of theories which can be divided further (see Chapter Seven, for example). However, for present purposes it is important to demonstrate just one thing: that it is incorrect to think of ethics as a single body of knowledge about right and wrong. Our social world is far more intricate and enigmatic than this.

## A DISTINCTION

We all, at one time or another, discuss moral issues. Such encounters happen daily: at work, in supermarket queues, in bars and public houses, on trains, at bus stops – everywhere where people are interested and concerned enough to discuss issues affecting human life and relationships. Typically, participants express their approval of various principles and argue that these should be followed by other people (sometimes they even follow them themselves). Most people's positions are not usually the result of thorough philosophical analysis, and from time to time we all advocate precepts that are either inconsistent with one another, or which contradict those for which we have argued previously. This unpredictability is acceptable at the level of casual conversation – it is all right in everyday ethics – but for another type of ethics – technical ethics – inconsistencies are usually studiously avoided.

## EVERYDAY ETHICS

The term 'everyday ethics' is not meant to be derogatory – indeed everyday ethical analysis is often more sincere than any other type. The term is used here to help clarify a difference in kind between largely unanalysed reactions to life situations and dilemmas (everyday ethics), and those grounded in more abstract, logical theory (technical ethics).

### One Example of Everyday Ethics

Different people's everyday ethics can vary immensely, both in content and consistency, and this can be a disadvantage if one is looking for clear thinking. Usually, in everyday ethics, only limited attention is paid to overall congruity, and it is common for everyday ethical decisions to be taken according to 'the moment' – according to the context and emotional state of a particular person at a particular time. Even for the same individual, different circumstances can give rise to different, even paradoxical, ethical intuitions. Consider, for example, the following possible 'system' of everyday ethics. This framework is one of an indefinite number of others – if all possible everyday ethical frameworks were to be incorporated into a 'grand vision' the contradictions and conflicts contained within would be mindboggling.

This particular everyday ethical outlook is based on a simple set of dictums. It is a crude framework which can give answers to some human problems, and it looks like this: 'sex before marriage is wrong', 'it is wrong to be underhand and deceitful at work', 'people who look after number one should be respected', 'you should always respect the wishes of other people', 'you should take only what a job is worth', 'adultery is acceptable so long as the adulterers are happy and no one gets hurt'.

There are problems even with this rudimentary ethic. For example, this everyday ethicist might be a neonatal nurse who respects an ambitious consultant (because he is very good at looking after number one). She discovers that the doctor is using robust physiotherapy experimentally on newborns, against the wishes of some of the parents (so she cannot respect everyone's wishes – the doctor wants to continue and the parents want her to stop him). Alternatively, the down-to-earth ethicist might be a bank employee who is a daily witness to an adulterous affair (which she thinks ethically acceptable) which necessitates deception in the workplace (which she considers not morally acceptable). It does not usually require too much investigation of any given everyday ethics to find contradiction – if a consistent ethical position is desired then something more than ad hoc frameworks and comfortable intuition is needed.

## TECHNICAL ETHICS

Technical ethics sets out to avoid the vagaries of everyday ethics, but has to pay a different price – technical ethicists sometimes have to sacrifice flexibility for the sake of coherence.

It is the job of moral philosophers to devise and refine technical ethical theory. They must design theories that are internally coherent, which contain principles and notions that complement each other, and which will enable those who act according to them to 'behave morally' (at least as that technical ethical theory defines 'moral') whatever the situation.

## ETHICS AND THE TIP OF THE ICEBERG

Technical ethics can be subdivided in various ways. Before some of these are explained it is necessary to offer a further clarification.

### A FURTHER DISTINCTION

A distinction can be made between **dramatic** or **specific ethics, persisting ethics**, and **ethics in a general sense**. This distinction is neither clear-cut nor wholly watertight. It breaks down when one sees the proper importance of the general sense of ethics, but it is nevertheless enlightening since it starts to explain why work for health must be seen as a moral endeavour. It can also help show how issues which seem ethically neutral are actually ethically vital, despite appearances.

(Note that it is well known amongst those who have failed to think up a less clichéd image that only the tips of icebergs are visible above the water.)

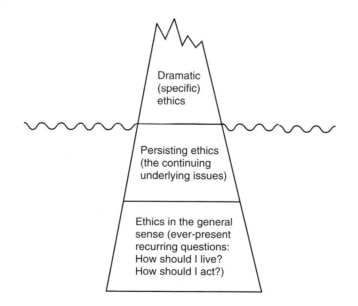

Dramatic
(specific)
ethics

Persisting ethics
(the continuing
underlying issues)

Ethics in the general
sense (ever-present
recurring questions:
How should I live?
How should I act?)

**Figure 9**   Ethics and the tip of the iceberg – a broad distinction between different types of ethics (not final or watertight)

## SPECIFIC OR DRAMATIC ETHICS

The term 'specific/dramatic ethics' (hereafter 'dramatic ethics') stands for the deliberation necessary when one is presented with a specific ethical problem – a matter that seems to stand self-contained, in isolation from other personal or work issues. Ethics in the dramatic sense is necessary when one is confronted with an obviously hard choice. For example, a doctor has a dramatic ethical problem when she wonders whether she ought to discontinue ventilation in order to transplant organs to three waiting recipients, all of whom stand a good chance of further fulfilling life, or whether she should continue treatment because of the slim possibility that a body might regain consciousness.

In this sort of dilemma a decision has to be made – one way or another. Having assessed the various pros and cons, all that is required is the courage to say – specifically – yes or no. Dramatic ethics is the domain of the 'tragic choice', where any choice bears a heavy cost. It is a place where – like it or not – one simply must fall into one camp or the other. Because dramatic ethical problems usually have lurid appeal, they tend to excite the makers of television documentaries. The consequent news-media focus on dramatic ethics has led to (or at least has reinforced) the now commonplace perception that such 'hot spots' are all there is to ethics. But they are really nothing more than ethics at the tip of the iceberg.

## PERSISTING ETHICS

As a result of sometimes rather facile media exposure 'persisting ethics' – the issues which permanently underlie the intermittent ethical dramas – has been underplayed. For example, behind the specific question: should abortion be a legal right? there are constant, philosophically fundamental questions about what it is to be a person or potential person, the degree of control a woman ought to have over what happens to her body, and the nature of a moral right.

## ETHICS IN THE GENERAL SENSE

The phrase 'ethics in the general sense' refers to deliberation – both abstract and concrete – about how best to conduct one's life in general. The person who deliberates in this general sense of ethics realises that moral questions are not only of occasional interest, but that all thought and all action can and should be the subject of moral reflection. Admittedly it might not be instantly obvious that decisions about whether or not to pass the salt to a fellow diner, or whether or not to continue sitting in an armchair doing nothing, have moral relevance, but they do in this general sense (see the discussion of *Ethical A and B* in the Introduction for a more complete explanation).

The basic point is that whatever one does, either to oneself or another, does not have to be done. Alternative courses of action are almost always possible, and these alternatives can have different consequences. Dependent upon what you choose to do, you can enhance or damage your own or someone else's existence.

To take the examples mentioned above: if you are asked to pass the salt at a dinner party you can do this gladly, casually, or with obvious irritation – possibly causing the person who made the request to feel more or less at ease. The result of a positive behaviour might be that the recipient will enjoy his meal more, be stimulated into interesting conversation, and you will probably have had a beneficial effect on all the diners. Alternatively, if you know something about nutrition and heart disease you might decide to inform your friend of the possible consequences of excessive salt consumption. You might tell him this nonchalantly, or jokingly, or seriously – you might even choose to scare him and cause him to feel guilty and anxious about his past habits.

And if you are sitting in an armchair you might be doing something else. In normal circumstances there should, of course, be no compulsion on a person not to sit in an armchair if that is what he chooses. However, the inescapable fact is that other things are possible. By remaining in the armchair (say you just happen to have woken up in it, you don't need to relax any more, and you simply continue to do nothing) you are doing little or nothing to create more of the possibilities open to yourself, nor are you doing anything to enable other people. It may not be the depth of immorality to remain in an armchair (everyone has got to be somewhere, after all) but neither is it the height of morality. You could be doing more. Whether or not to sit in an armchair is a moral issue.

## TWO ILLUSTRATIONS OF THE ICEBERG DISTINCTIONS

1. The 1982 conflict – fast becoming a distant memory – between Great Britain and Argentina over the Falkland Islands (or Malvinas) gives an especially clear picture of the tip of the iceberg phenomenon. The conflict flared quickly and was soon over. It focused intense interest in some quarters on dramatic ethical issues. There was, for instance, widespread discussion about the morality of killing hundreds of people over a relatively barren and sparsely populated island; about whether the principle of 'sovereignty' should take precedence over the principle of 'common humanity'; about whether Britain has a clear and certain duty to protect her citizens wherever, and in whatever circumstances, they might be; and about whether blatant lying and secrecy, by a democratically elected government in 'communication' with the general public is ethically correct even in time of war.

   Although these *dramatic* ethical issues are no longer in the limelight, they remain at the iceberg's summit. But lying below the water, at the next level down, are *persisting* ethical questions which existed before, during, and after the Falklands conflict. These are at least as important as the dramatic ones, even though they are not so immediately apparent. They include such questions as: Is it moral to maintain a large army in peace time when the social and environmental conditions of millions of British citizens are self-evidently debilitating? Should the public have access to more information about the workings of the military? Should pacifists have the right to refuse to pay taxation to maintain armed forces? Should governments elected by a minority of votes have the right to call upon everyone to go to war?

   Ethics in the *general sense* is depicted at the base of the iceberg in Figure 9, but in truth it permeates the whole edifice. Yet it is hard for us to see life like this, and so we rarely focus on ethics in the general sense. We become aware of this part of the iceberg only when we think of ethics as a personal task, as we do when we ask such questions as 'What can I do about these dramatic and persisting issues?' 'Should I campaign to put over my point of view?' 'Should I distort evidence to persuade people of my position?' 'If I am with a group of relative strangers, perhaps in a pub after a few drinks, all of whom vehemently support a position to which I am strongly opposed, should I explain what I believe or should I let it pass?' Such questions are no less hard to answer than those raised in the rest of the iceberg. Indeed, they can be the hardest of all.

2. Because ethics in the general sense is such a feature of human life (like the air we breathe) we tend not to realise that we are constantly faced with ethical situations: as a rule we do not examine most of what we do. Once we become aware of the extent of ethics in a general sense we recognise the true magnitude of our responsibilities – and this can be such an overwhelming discovery that still we do not face up to them. We would, of course, be made insane if we reflected ethically on everything, nor can anyone do very much about most of life's injustices – not even those which trouble us greatly. However, to know ethics in the general sense is constantly to be aware of the tension between duty and inertia – a tension between doing what one ought to, and going along with things as they are.

As I write this second edition I am more acutely aware than ever how easy it is to shirk responsibility, even though I know I *must* ask myself 'How should I act?' 'How should I live?' 'What should I do for the moral best?' I am a lecturer in a medical school, and have had the job for long enough to have a list as long as my arm of all that is not right – and yet I do nothing very much about it, justifying my policy on utilitarian grounds (I tell myself it is better in general that I'm around to teach the undergraduates).

Just from everyday observation, I know of many patients who are being treated shabbily yet I usually do nothing to help them. I continually come across dramatic ethical issues (most commonly – patients not being properly informed of their conditions, not for resuscitation notes placed almost arbitrarily, and rationing decisions made covertly, according to social and ethnic criteria) each of which raises central, persisting questions. I know, from what I understand of ethics in the general sense, that it is not enough to shrug – to say, it is too big for me, what can I do? – for I could do all sorts of things if I wanted to. But I do not because I'm sure the consequences are unlikely to be good for me, or for the reputation of ethics teaching where I work.

I am currently deeply troubled by a patient who has been kept in a secure mental illness unit for two years. The circumstances which led to her incarceration were certainly *dramatic* – she was arrested and accused of repeated intimidation, she screamed her protests in the cells, she was committed involuntarily for psychiatric treatment, she was diagnosed 'erotomanic' (amongst other things), she thinks she is a witch, and she has since consistently failed to respond to treatment in the ways her medical guardians want (she will not, for instance, agree that she is or ever has been mentally ill).

The *persisting* issues are far too numerous to list fully, though they include questions about the nature of mental illness, psychiatric taxonomy, the point of involuntary treatment (is it to cure, to restrain or to protect?), competence (the patient is extremely clear about what has happened to her), the relationship between criminal responsibility and insanity, the motivations of psychiatrists, and the clash between cultural outlooks (her family and her ancestors are witches too).

*Ethics in the general sense* requires me to consider how best to act in this case. Should I do nothing, should I work subtly behind the scenes by speaking with her psychiatrists – most of whom I know a little, should I advocate for her more openly, or should I try to publicise her case in the press? Whatever I do I know this is not only an issue for her – it is an ethical issue for me too.

## ASPECTS OF TECHNICAL ETHICS

Technical ethics can be divided into various aspects. Different analysts have devised many different classifications. Three of these – *moral philosophy as a quest to understand 'the good', moral philosophy based on either consequences or duties, and moral philosophy as a process of deliberation* – may be particularly illuminating for students of health care ethics.

### I.   MORAL PHILOSOPHY AS A QUEST TO UNDERSTAND 'THE GOOD'

One branch of technical ethics does not aim to tackle ethical problems directly, although this may ultimately be a consequence. Instead this form seeks to understand the nature of 'goodness' since (it is argued) it is only by first understanding what goodness means that anyone can aim to be good.

It is possible to become so preoccupied with questions of meaning that it is only meaning – and nothing else – that is seen as the problem. So, two points need to be restated. Firstly, it is crucial, in any serious inquiry, that the meanings of key terms are clarified as far as possible. But secondly, it must not be thought that real problems can be solved merely by clarifying the meanings of words. The clarification of meaning is an essential part of inquiry into ethics, but it is only a part.

### Good

For example, in order to work out what it is good to do it is important to stress that the word 'good' has at least three separate meanings.

a. *'Good' as a description of objects that are useful*
   People talk of a 'good clock' or a 'good motor car' using this sense of 'good'. Used in this way 'good' is often ethically neutral, at least when it is used to describe a physical function *per se* (this is a good clock because it tells the time accurately, which is what it is supposed to do: this is a good car because I can rely on it to start in the morning). Of course, if one asks: what is this good (functionally efficient) car being used for? then one is asking for an answer with moral content. For example, the car might be being used by a volunteer to transport disabled people to Day Centres, or it might be a getaway car for armed robbers, and there is normally a moral difference between these two purposes.

b. *'Good' as a description of things that are pleasing or enjoyable in themselves*
Using 'good' in this sense it is possible to describe an aesthetically pleasing painting, or a productive garden, as good in an ethically neutral way – though even used like this it is not implausible to argue that there is ethical content nevertheless (see the Introduction).

c. *'Good' used to describe the specifically moral*
When the word 'good' is used like this it describes human activity – usually human activity that affects other people, not only the actor. This use of the word has close connections with other moral words such as 'ought', 'right', 'just', and 'duty'. It is frequently asserted, for instance, that a person ought to do what is good.

## 2.   MORAL PHILOSOPHY BASED ON EITHER CONSEQUENCES OR DUTIES

A central controversy in moral philosophy stems from the possibility of thinking of ethics in two apparently very different ways: basing decisions about how to act on the assessment of the likely consequences of those actions, and basing decisions about how to act on moral duties.

By way of introduction to this pivotal debate – which is enlarged in Chapter Seven – consider these traditional examples.

### Consequences

One technical ethical theory is known as utilitarianism. Generally speaking, utilitarians assess the morality of people's actions either by looking at the actual results (and so judging morality in retrospect) or by calculating likely future outcomes. For utilitarians the best (most moral) actions are those which produce the most favourable balance of good over bad. So the worth of any action – whether it is a small kindness to another person, or a decision to declare war on a nation – is considered to be moral or immoral dependent on whether or not the outcome is a balance of human happiness over misery (at least according to one version of utilitarianism).

### Duties

The competing version of technical ethics is deontology. Generally speaking, according to this outlook what matters most is not the result but the fact that a person acted according to a perceived duty. For example, an advocate of deontology might argue that certain principles, truth-telling and promise-keeping perhaps, are fundamental to morality and that, to be moral, a person has an obligation always to abide by them – whatever the consequences. Even if the outcome of telling the truth will produce more misery than happiness, to tell it – to abide by preconceived moral duty – is the right and honest way to act.

## 3.   MORAL PHILOSOPHY AS A PROCESS OF DELIBERATION

This form of technical ethics is different from the types identified so far because it makes an ultimate plea neither to rules nor to past and future consequences. This variety – moral philosophy as a deliberative process – is the type developed and espoused in this book, and is perhaps closest to the Aristotelian view of ethics. This variant of technical ethics has two key aspects: *the process* of deliberation and its *goal*.

*The process* is not a blind or chance procedure. If the reasoning is to have depth the thinker must have a grasp of a number of principles and methods, as well as a sense of balance and personal maturity. The aim of the process advocated in this book (and captured in the Ethical Grid) is human flourishing: the most fundamental form of morality possible. The idea is that the most moral endeavours are those which aim to produce as much enhancing human potential as possible, as much of what human beings are for as can be achieved.

The general nature of this goal can be indicated, simplistically for now, in the following way. It is contained in the very nature of an acorn that it can become an oak tree. In order for the acorn to achieve this potential it must go through a number of stages of development successfully, the environmental conditions must be conducive to its proper development, and no serious obstacles must impede its growth (for the acorn and growing oak these obstacles might include lumberjacks, drought, fires, diseases, locusts, and town planners). In a like, though vastly more complicated and unpredictable way, it is in the nature of a day-old child to become a uniquely fulfilled adult dependent upon personal and external conditions.

The essence of deliberative ethics is consideration of the best ways to create more of what might be in oneself and others. This version of moral reasoning is difficult to master for those who believe that being ethical is a question of following specific rules and codes of conduct, or of always acting according to a specific view of what is right and wrong.

Aristotle thought deliberation was the essence of ethics, since a contemplative process must be undertaken in every case where there are conclusions to be reached about the worth of human activity. He divided knowledge into three different disciplines: theoretical, practical, and productive.[30] The majority of his works were concerned with his 'theoretical' category: 'natural science' – where 'natural and regular laws' apply. According to Aristotle, there is no need for deliberation under this heading because this is the realm of fact, of mathematical law, and of predictable physical cause and effect.

But ethics is different. In ethical matters there is not the certainty of natural science. Rather there is an indefinite – perhaps even infinite – variety of human circumstances and situations, and there can be no universal laws or sets of principles that can be applied to every situation. Whatever rule is invented in moral philosophy, sooner or later there will be a case in which it will be better to break it in order to create a better human potential. And because of this it is far better – far more moral – to enhance human judgement in the uncertain field of human action and interaction, rather than to instil imperfect sets of rules in people, as if these rules are inviolable commandments. Rules and principles are useful to the deliberative process, but subjective judgement in context is ultimate.

## ETHICS AND HEALTH WORKERS

Many health workers have not, until recently, had the opportunity to appreciate the enlightening distinctions made by good moral philosophy. Many can still see nothing more than the tip of the iceberg, yet it is only by discovering all its contours that health workers can bring about the best new paradigm. Health workers should not be blamed for their lack of awareness because:

1. They receive very limited, or even no formal training in ethics, even though their daily work involves direct and often crucial intervention in other people's lives.
2. Health workers usually have urgent practical jobs which allow them little time to pause for thought. Furthermore, there is little provision within traditional health services for classes and discussion groups to enable health workers to reflect more deeply on the ethics of their endeavours.
3. Many books on ethics speak in a language and manner which most health workers find alien (numerous examples of such books can be found on library shelves between the Dewey classifications 170–174 or Library of Congress reference BJ). Although health work begets interesting cases by the hour, the examples given to illustrate moral theory in these books are frequently artificial and hypothetical. And if real cases are used – as is the fashion in contemporary 'bioethics' – they are almost always dramatic – and so equally if not more misleading than the imaginary ones.

## PROGRESS SO FAR

It was argued in Chapter One that there is an intellectual crisis in health care, and that its future form depends both upon which theories of health come to dominate and how present health workers choose to intervene in their clients' lives. It was contended that the most desirable future – the best new paradigm – may be created once health workers better understand the nature of ethics, and once they recognise the implications of the slogan 'work for health is a moral endeavour'.

Further points and clarifications have been made in Chapter Two:

1. Work for health is a moral endeavour because work for health can release more or less human potential. Roughly speaking, the more enhancing potentials liberated, the higher the degree of morality produced by an intervention.
2. Ethics is a complex field, not merely a means of deciding between clear-cut rights and wrongs.
3. Enlightening distinctions can be made between everyday ethics and technical ethics, and between dramatic ethics, persisting ethics, and ethics in the general sense.
4. Technical ethics can be divided into different aspects. Ethics as deliberation is the aspect preferred in this book since it emphasises both process and aim and is based on the notion of ethics in the general sense.

# CHAPTER THREE

# Uncovering the Basic Questions

It appears to me that in Ethics as in all other philosophical studies, the difficulties and disagreements, of which its history is full, are mainly due to a very simple cause: namely to the attempt to answer questions, without firstly discovering precisely what question it is which you desire to answer.[31]

## WHAT IS THE KEY QUESTION FOR HEALTH WORKERS?

What question should health workers be asking? Which question – once properly answered – will bring about the new paradigm? Modern health workers face a multitude of dramatic, persisting and general ethical questions, but none of them is fundamental (the dramatic ones least of all). Instead – unlikely as it may seem at first – the general key question is this: *what is the relationship between morality and work for health?*

Health work, in its most complete sense, is work aimed at preventing or eliminating obstacles that might or do stand in the way of individuals' biological and chosen potentials (so long as the achievement of these potentials causes no intentional harm to other human beings). And just as this is the true nature of work for health so it is also the true nature of moral endeavour, at least where ethics is understood to be a process of deliberation about how best to act in the presence of other lives.

What is the point of mending a broken leg? What is the point of helping a person overcome emotional trauma through counselling? What is the point of trying to cure cancer? What is the point of attempting to enable a cancer sufferer come to terms with his illness, and to accept the new limitations of his existence? Surely the point is to enable each person to achieve more of whatever potential she has to live a fulfilled life. The point of eliminating obstacles to potential is not just that we judge the obstacles undesirable *per se*, the point is to get rid of them in order to release the good they are blocking.

## A VITAL LINK

To spell it out further: the fundamental link between health work and morality is this. Whatever health is taken to mean, work for health has to involve intervention in human lives. That it is possible to make a difference to people's lives – for better or worse – is also the key to the importance of morality: moral philosophers are concerned about human thought and action because, and in so far as, this has social implications.

In work for health a range of types of intervention are possible – all of which naturally have moral implications. Consider, for instance, the rather mundane example of setting and mending a broken wrist (any other health intervention example would serve equally well as an illustration).

## TWO SITUATIONS

1. *The first situation*

A young man has been playing soccer and, during a hopelessly optimistic attempt at an overhead kick, has landed awkwardly and broken his left wrist. He does not know he has a broken bone but is in great pain and so visits the casualty department. On reporting to reception he is told in an unfriendly way to sit and wait his turn. He asks how long he will have to wait, but the receptionist tells him she has no idea. He then eats a packetful of boiled sweets. Three quarters of an hour later he is approached by a nurse who conducts him to a small windowless room in which the doctor is sitting. The doctor does not look directly at the young man but focuses on the wrist, which he examines. He mumbles a few questions and then sends the patient to X-ray. The young man asks whether the bone is broken, and whether he need be in such pain. The doctor just shrugs, and tells him not to be a baby.

The X-ray shows that the bone is broken and needs to be reset. A nurse arrives then and – in order to see whether or not it will be safe to administer a general anaesthetic – she asks the young man whether he has eaten anything during the last 12 hours. He replies that all he has eaten is a bagful of boiled sweets, to which the nurse says sorry, all she can do is administer a local anaesthetic.

The anaesthetic is duly given and the young man told to wait fifteen minutes for the pain to stop. But it persists. The young man informs the doctor of this just as he is about to take him into a side room to set the wrist. The doctor expresses surprise, but reluctantly agrees to wait a further fifteen minutes.

Still the pain persists, and by now the young man is becoming anguished and fearful. He tells the doctor he is still in as much pain as ever, but the doctor does not believe him and, ignoring his protests, begins to set the wrist. This causes the patient excruciating agony. He screams involuntarily and is held down by three nurses until the doctor has done his work. After further pain and screams the doctor is satisfied. Without a word to the young man – of either explanation or apology – he leaves and a plaster cast is placed on the wrist by a surly technician. An appointment is made for the young man to return in two days' time, to check that the broken bone is still in the right place. He is advised to take paracetamol for the pain and to rest. Nothing else.

2. *An alternative*

The same young man has been playing football and, during the same ludicrous execution of an overhead kick, has broken his left wrist. He visits the casualty department. On reporting to reception he is treated with kindness and sympathy.

The receptionist, noting that the young man appears to be suffering a degree of shock (from the result of his injury rather than from any surprise at having played soccer so miserably), asks him how he is feeling and would he like to call anyone, and then invites him to sit and wait for the nurse, who will attend him as soon as she has seen patients who arrived before him – this will probably be in half an hour or so. The receptionist asks the young man whether he has eaten or drunk for the last 12 hours (it is now around mid-afternoon) and he replies that his last meal was supper yesterday. The receptionist explains that in this case it is best that he not eat anything now since it might just be that he will need a general anaesthetic, but that there is nothing at all to be alarmed about.

The nurse arrives and takes the young man to the doctor, who examines the wrist without causing pain. As he thinks, the doctor explains in non-technical language what he believes might have happened. The likelihood is that the wrist is broken, but to be sure and to enable the bone to be set most effectively it will be necessary to take X-rays.

The X-ray confirms the bone is broken and, after checking that the man has not eaten for nearly 24 hours, and after carefully explaining exactly what will happen to him and to his arm, and how he can expect to feel when he comes round, and after gaining the young man's permission, the doctor organises the administration of a general anaesthetic. The bone is set.

When he regains consciousness a nurse sits with him until he feels well enough for his friend to drive him home. She explains about the visits he will have to make to the hospital in the future, about how quickly the pain will subside, and about how soon he could expect to play football again (not that this is a major anxiety after his last effort). He is given paracetamol for the pain, and asked whether he drinks or smokes cannabis. He says that he is fond of a drink and the nurse tells him that in this case a drink will probably do as well as the paracetamol, but he should not take both together, which would be dangerous.

## WHAT DO THESE TWO SITUATIONS INDICATE?

These situations go some way toward establishing the claim that work for health is a moral endeavour. They show that even in apparently routine health interventions – in everyday work for health – the manner in which a person is treated (and health produced) is inevitably bound up with the degree of morality created. Each of the health workers involved in the two situations was responsible for intervening in another person's life. And although setting bones is an everyday procedure for some health workers it was a time of crisis for the young man.

All the health workers involved had a degree of choice about what they did. They were bound by contracts of employment, and may have wished to conform to professional codes of practice, but even within these boundaries (which as autonomous individuals they could choose to accept or not) a range of personal behaviour was possible. Quite different physical, emotional and intellectual consequences could have been experienced by the young man, dependent upon how the health workers chose to act.

These observations will be familiar to most people concerned about their responsibilities to others. How each of us should behave towards our fellow beings is the central ethical question. If anything it is of greatest importance in health work, which has the express purpose of helping the vulnerable.

This conclusion follows. By its very nature health work is intentional intervention in the lives of other people. These interventions are made either directly – by a caring touch, by the surgeon's knife, in the consultation, by face to face education – or indirectly – by the hospital administrator deciding which ward to close, by the government ministers agreeing a health service budget, by the manager implementing a new nutrition policy, or by the supervisor deciding upon the best working conditions for staff. Whether these interventions are made directly or indirectly, at some point they have real – often major – implications for human lives.

## THE SPECIFIC KEY QUESTION

The basic challenge for any health worker, in each case and in general, is to work out how to make the best possible moral intervention.

Therefore, the key question for health workers is '*How can I intervene to the highest moral degree?*' This question unites work for health with morality. It should be the permanent starting point for all health work.

Unfortunately, though this key question can be inspiring, it is so general that it is uninformative. For some people 'being ethical' means always conforming to a particular view about what is right and wrong. But when two people hold conflicting opinions about right and wrong in particular circumstances (as often happens) then their choices will conflict. Different people can have divergent ideas about how to intervene to the highest moral degree.

Considering that all involved are supposed to be working for health, such conflict is remarkably common in medicine. For example, some doctors take the view that it is unquestionably right to abort a foetus if this is the pregnant woman's choice, while others think it morally repugnant to destroy something that has the potential to become a competent human being. Some doctors take the view that heroic resuscitations are morally required to save severely handicapped neonates, while others think this policy cruel for all concerned. In cases such as these it seems futile to advise health workers to think about how to intervene to the most moral degree. In such contexts morality seems relative and contestable – the competing views irreconcilable, and the idea of intervening morally open to almost any interpretation.

But this is not necessarily so. While it is a fact of life that people often hold different values, which sometimes lead them to make different choices in their interventions with others, it is nevertheless possible – given that the essence of morality is the act of deliberating with integrity – to be clear that some interventions in the name of health are of a higher moral calibre than others.

Consider again the two situations above. In both cases effort aimed at creating health in the young man produced some degree of morality. The way to work out which behaviours generated the highest degree of morality is to note the extent to which the various aspects of the young man, thought of as a person rather than merely as a human body with a broken wrist, were repaired, enhanced, or developed.

Even in the down-to-earth setting of a casualty department there were opportunities to carry out very different sorts of intervention. In both situations the wrist was set. But in the first it was fixed with great and unnecessary pain, and the young man suffered uncertainty and anxiety: partly as a result of the receptionist's failure to inform him not to eat the boiled sweets, partly because he was not listened to by other staff, and because nothing of significance was explained to him. In the second situation attention was paid to his physical comfort, and time spent to enable him to understand his temporarily disabled circumstances and the future development of his wrist. He was also helped to feel emotionally calm and generally safe.

In the first case the young man was enabled in a physical sense, but there was no attempt to enable him to understand or be reassured, and there was no intention – no need seen – to respect his opinions, feelings, or wishes. The idea seems to have been that these were either irrelevant, wrong or both. In the second situation the wrist was set, and here too the man was enabled physically. But in this case he was also educated, his immediate emotional needs were detected and addressed, and he was treated with respect. He was asked to choose after options were explained to him.

It is surely not unreasonable to conclude provisionally, even without the argument of the remainder of this book, that the interventions which took place in the second situation were of a higher moral standard than those which took place in the first (competent use of the Ethical Grid will indicate how such a position might be justified).

## OTHER IMPORTANT QUESTIONS AND TOPICS

The identification of the central question for health work is only part of the initial task. The cardinal question for health workers – 'How can I intervene to the highest moral degree?' – is not a catch-all, nor is it always the most appropriate question to ask, but it provides orientation to other questions thoughtful health workers must consider.

## CENTRAL TOPICS

The chief priority for any serious inquiry is to ensure its questions are of the highest relevance. By posing the right questions it becomes possible to grasp the soul of a problem.

The central areas of concern are these:

1. *How can we work to create more health when we do not:*
   a. know for certain what health is?
   b. agree between ourselves what health is?
   These questions still need to be asked, though strong answers have now been proposed[1,5] as a result of practical philosophical analysis. By focusing primarily on

the moral content of work for health it is hoped that this book will make agreement about the nature of health, and the limits to work for health, more likely still.

2. *How can we be ethical when we do not:*

   a. know for certain what it is to be ethical?

   b. agree between ourselves what it is to be ethical?

   These questions are of vital importance for this analysis. Without proper clarification of the nature of ethics, without a clear idea of the different possible ethical understandings it is impossible to reach any decision about the morality of interventions. And practically speaking, without explication of the limits of morality, there can be no end to the actions people might justify as moral.

3. *The nature of interventions*

   a. *What is an intervention? What types of intervention are there?*

   It is possible to distinguish various types of intervention. For example, there are clear differences of kind and moral implication between:

      i. An intervention requested and agreed to. For example, when a man voluntarily consults his general practitioner.

      ii. An intervention that is not requested but which the client desires, or finds desirable. For example, when a health visitor or district nurse calls unannounced and finds an old lady alone without heating, and too proud to ask for help.

      iii. An intervention neither requested nor desired. For example, when a health professional visits the house of a smoker unasked to tell him why he should stop. Or when a consultant undertakes controlled tests on groups of patients without their knowledge (and which they would not want to be part of, given the choice).

      iv. An intervention enforced by law. Examples in this category include interventions to quarantine people with notifiable diseases, compulsory sterilisation of women defined as mentally subnormal, and interventions to detain persons under Mental Health Acts.

      v. Not intervening, through neglect. For example, when a social worker fails to notice signs of child abuse.

      vi. Radical non-intervention. Sometimes, in social work for instance, decisions are taken not to intervene where interventions would normally be made, on the ground that the physical risk to the worker is too great.

   b. *In what ways can interventions be justified?*

   The intention of the person who is to intervene, and the predicted and actual consequences of the intervention have to be considered if the morality of the intervention is to be assessed. For example, it might be argued that the degree of morality exhibited by a consultant testing physiotherapy on neonates without their parents' knowledge, will vary dependent on her motive and the potential or actual benefits and dangers.

   c. *What is the difference (if any) between an intervention that raises ethical issues and an intervention that does not?*

   It is often thought that there is a clear difference between interventions with a moral dimension and those that are morally neutral. But as this book shows, this distinction cannot be sustained (see the Introduction for more on this).

4. *How can a clear limit to health interventions be set out* (there must be one if the expression 'health intervention' is meaningful)? How can this limit be informative

and useful without imposing rigid rules and codes on health workers? As we shall see, the Ethical Grid offers one answer to this question.

5. *What is a person? What is a full person?* This is a central topic too. Thinking about what we mean by the word 'person' helps make it clear why we should respect other people. It helps clarify why we bother to work for health at all, and why ethical analysis can be so civilising.

It is possible to distinguish between 'a person in a basic sense' and 'full persons'. Work for health is work to ensure that there are more full persons in the world.

## THE STAGE IS SET

The problem has been outlined. Health workers must find a way to ensure that future health care is of the best possible kind. A path towards an answer has been sketched out: understanding ethics can provide the key.

Initial distinctions have been made, and a central question identified. The stage is set for case studies to be presented, for the inquiry proper to begin, and for a means of coping with problems of practice to be offered.

# CHAPTER FOUR

# Problems of Practice

## INTRODUCTION

Theoretically informed, practical solutions to the question: what ought to be done in health care's name? require systematic critical analysis. To arrive consistently at high-quality answers takes practice. But given an understanding of ethical reasoning and how to do it health workers' analytic skills can be greatly improved by regular exercise on real-world cases.

The case studies and questions set out in this chapter offer an initial intellectual workout. Doing them is unlikely to turn practitioners into first class ethical analysts overnight but the exercises should be attempted at this stage of the book nonetheless, in order to show (if further proof be needed) that some form of ethical analysis is indispensable in health work. Ideally, each exercise should be revisited with the aid of the Ethical Grid (see Chapter Ten), once this instrument has been studied.

Given that a major theme of this book is that the present focus of health work is limited by overemphasis on the elimination and prevention of disease and illness, it might appear strange that all fifteen case studies described here have to do with disease and illness. However, there are four reasons for sticking with conventional case studies in preference to, say, exercises about education or the distribution of warm and safe housing. These are:

1. The studies have relevance and interest for present health workers.
2. Medical work against disease and illness can be a genuine part of work for health, and will obviously remain so.
3. The paradigm change is in progress. The studies help show that within present health work there are elements of the fading paradigm and the new era.
4. By focusing on current health work practice, and by showing that a richer theory of health needs to be widely acknowledged, it might be possible to accelerate the paradigm change.

None of the case studies has an obviously right answer. There are always alternative courses of action – often several – open to the participants in each study. Any of them will require justification. Why this solution and not another one?

When attempting to tackle each problem it will be productive for any interested reader to write down the course of action she would take or advise, together with her reasons and any criticisms of rejected options. Alternatively she might simply write down her feelings and intuitions about the cases. It may be enlightening for her to consider later, when the nature of ethics and the reasoning behind various ethical theories has been explained in more detail, whether her understanding of her proposals has been enlarged. It might even be that her thinking will have changed as a result. If so this will be a welcome success for applied philosophy.

# THE CASE STUDIES

Every case study raises an assortment of issues, not all of which will be immediately apparent. Tasks are suggested, at the foot of each study, for those readers who wish to begin to explore the moral issues independently or in groups.

## I.   TEACHING OR CARING: MICHAEL AND CAROLINE

Michael is a health visitor, devoted to his profession. He feels it allows him to do professionally what he would wish to do voluntarily anyway. He believes passionately that the primary reason for any person's existence is to help others.

A sensitive man who empathises naturally with nearly everyone he meets, Michael lives to care. He has the gift of seeing life as other people see it. He can shift easily into the attitudes of those he looks after. Michael often says that the secret of good health visiting is 'to be able to step temporarily into the other person's shoes'. The trouble – if indeed it is trouble – is that some of his many friends worry that sometimes Michael's temporary becomes a little too permanent.

The seeds of this situation were sown during Michael's time as a student health visitor. An incident which happened at the end of his training upset him profoundly, so much so that he was unable to articulate fully all the aspects which distressed him. As part of his fieldwork experience Michael was assigned an elderly lady to visit once a month, between October and June. Caroline was 79, a widow, rather frail but still able to cook and clean. She had a home help twice a week. She did not suffer from any disease as far as anyone knew, and the only medication she needed was a good sized tumbler of neat whisky every evening.

Caroline could reflect on a rich life. She had married twice, once to a journalist and then – several years after her divorce – to a successful businessman. She had been able to travel widely with both her husbands, meeting an enormous variety of people on the way, and had written about her experiences in two books. Her problem now was loneliness. Her husband had died three years ago, and she still missed him desperately.

Michael did not see his health visiting role from a medical perspective. Indeed, his brief was simply to observe and support Caroline. He did not consider himself primarily a nurse (he was basically supposed to make sure Caroline did not suffer physical illness and injury) even though he accepted that this is an important role for health visitors in many contexts. Rather Michael felt his role was to befriend the widow, to help her see the past with fondness instead of regret and longing, to help her focus on the talents and possibilities that still remained open to her, and to encourage her to share herself with other people.

_ continues _

*continued*

Over the months Michael and Caroline became friends, despite the 45 year age gap. Though the process had been slow, Caroline had begun to think about what she could do now rather than what she had done in the past. As for Michael, he was pleased with what he was achieving with Caroline, and he too had developed. Caroline had built up a hard edge, a cynicism, during her dealings with people in journalism and business. Her stories, her accounts of her decisions and of the politics of life, saddened the committed altruist, but he recognised a certain truth in what she was saying, a necessity about what she had done. Michael was benefiting too.

Then, for reasons his superior refused to outline, Michael was assigned a different case load when he qualified, even though he was still operating the same 'patch' as before. Michael explained that he believed he was doing useful work with Caroline, and what was more he was enjoying it and thought it right to continue. But all his supervisor would say was that the old lady's circumstances did not merit the services of a busy health visitor. She was, she had to say, useful only as part of the 'learning experience'. Michael said that in that case he would continue to visit Caroline in a private capacity, but his supervisor replied curtly that this would not be advisable. It would be unprofessional behaviour.

## *EXERCISE*

Write out the key issues as they occur to you.

State your approval or disapproval of any of the interventions made in this study.

Suggest ways in which things could be done differently (by any of the characters), in order to achieve a higher degree of morality.

Explain what you take 'higher degree of morality' to mean.

As far as you can, justify your opinions and suggestions.

## 2. TELLING THE TRUTH?

Two health education officers, Barbara and Kim, have been instructed to launch a campaign to improve local people's diets. They work in a small department managed by a district health education officer. The department is based in an inner-city area in the north-west of England, and the two officers are familiar with its high unemployment, avoidable disease, and general deprivation. Both Barbara and Kim are Social Science graduates, well-equipped to research their subject area.

The District Medical Officer, who manages the District Health Education Officer and makes policy decisions, has instructed that the campaign must be based solely on the guidelines presented in a recently published booklet.

*continues*

continued

Barbara and Kim consider what to do. Kim decides almost immediately that she must, as a responsible and professional health education officer, carry out her orders to the letter. But Barbara has several worries.

Barbara has concerns about the following aspects of the campaign. First, she has found out that the costs of publishing the booklet were born equally by the Health Education Authority and the butter industry. Secondly, Barbara has come to the conclusion that although the booklet is sumptuously produced – colourful, graphic, and glossy – it is very hard to read. In fact it is far from clear what the practical advice is. Barbara wonders whether it is possible the information has been presented in this way deliberately in order to confuse, so that people stick with their present habits. She cannot be sure of the intentions of the writers and artists, but is worried about the effects the booklet might have. Thirdly, from her research she has learnt that some of the information (in this case especially about fats) is significantly incomplete, to the extent that a biased picture appears to have been presented. Fourthly, Barbara is not at all sure that the information and advice – the 'nutrition facts' – given in the booklet are necessarily the truth. Much of it seems to be opinion rather than certainty. To expound opinion in the guise of fact seems to Barbara to be propaganda, and she does not want to be involved in a brainwashing exercise.

Barbara has spent time exploring the history of nutrition research and advice and realises that much depends upon the fashions of the time, the social trends of a particular era, the types of foods available, and the amount of money people have to spend on food. She has also read alternative theories to those presented in the booklet, and knows that informed commentators dispute several of the booklet's claims. Furthermore, when the social nature of the area is taken into account it is questionable whether or not the campaign will be effective. It could turn out to be a waste of time and money. People living in nearby tower blocks, in damp, noisy, crowded conditions, unable to find work, and under considerable pressure from life's iniquitous burdens are unlikely to change the comforting habits of a lifetime because of glossy advice delivered by a pair of reasonably well-off, middle-class health education officers.

Barbara explains her worries and findings to Kim, who listens and understands Barbara's point of view, but none the less insists on doing her duty as a health education officer working for the health service. She can, she says, hardly do anything other than defer to the opinion of a qualified medic.

## EXERCISE

Write out the key issues as they occur to you.

In your opinion, which of the health education officers is attempting to intervene with the highest degree of morality?

What should Barbara do? How might she behave in this situation in order to achieve the highest degree of morality as she understands it?

As far as you can, justify your opinions and suggestions.

## 3. TO IMMUNISE OR NOT?

Diane is a health visitor employed by a Health Authority responsible for the health of 5 million citizens. The Authority is chaired by an ambitious man, and has an uncompromising policy on immunisation and vaccination. The chairman is determined that his district will return the best vaccination figures in the country. He sees the task as a sales campaign and each employee as an agent for the policy – as a sales representative, in other words. An aggressive policy is also strongly advocated by the Specialist in Community Medicine (Child Health). Various pressures have been brought to bear on all local general practitioners to ensure they are as effective as possible in the campaign, but it is the health visitors who are seen as the main 'message-bearers' since it is possible for them to exert direct pressure on clients – on mothers whose children are due for immunisation. Such phrases as 'go on, it's the right thing to do', 'you really must agree, all the other mums have', 'it's much safer than not vaccinating', 'I've had all mine done' and 'it's only fair on the child, you know' can be very powerful when said by professionals to women who are uncertain what to do, lack the means to research the pros and cons for themselves, and want the best for their children.

The Authority's target is a straightforward 100% uptake for all those who show no contra-indications. The main thrust of the present campaign is set against whooping cough. The health visitors have been instructed to convince every parent or guardian of each child visited that the vaccination is *definitely* in the interest of each child. But Diane has doubts. She has researched the subject and, against the current tide of opinion, has arrived at the view that the risks of immunisation outweigh the benefits[32,33] and that this is what the campaign ought to be saying, while at the same time offering the service to those who wish it. Diane knows that she would not choose to have her child vaccinated, and so she cannot honestly advocate vaccination.

Diane decides firstly that she is not prepared to run the risk of directly inflicting injury upon another human being. She would prefer instead to make sure that each child is fit, well housed, and well nourished, and so better able to cope with whooping cough if it strikes. Secondly, Diane is opposed to a high-pressure sales campaign because she is not prepared to frighten another person unnecessarily, or to inflict stress and guilt upon someone who refuses to cooperate.

Diane's problem is that as a professional working for the State she has a contractual duty to follow the instructions she has been given. If she fails to do so she must accept possible dismissal, and even legal action, if a parent can show that Diane gave false or misleading information. Yet as an individual in her own right, as a person with opinions she feels she can justify, Diane believes she should not obey the Health Authority's command. She believes the campaign is deceitful and probably dangerous, and that less overall benefit will result from it than from her preferred policy.

Diane thinks the true hub of the issue is not actually to do with whether it is better to immunise or not. The evidence for and against is uncertain, and there are risks associated with vaccination that no one can honestly deny. Given this uncertainty Diane perceives that what is at stake is how people treat others. She is, she believes, being asked to lie, to coerce, and to treat adults as if they are children who can cope only with simplicities and one side of the story. She does not wish to be party to what she regards as a mass insult against the local people, even one genuinely intended to be for the good of the population as a whole. What is good is arguable, and Diane thinks there are a number of possible candidates for the title 'supreme good' in this case. Among these are the notions of respect for fellow persons, and regarding and treating other people as intellectually valuable and autonomous, or potentially autonomous. Diane casts these goods, on this occasion, above the good of possibly preventing physical harm.

*continues*

_ continued _

Diane also takes into account the fact that middle-class children are vaccinated to raise herd immunity, although those children are not in personal need of it.[33] This is never explained to their parents for fear they might refuse, even though it would be far more respectful and honest for the advocates of childhood immunisation to ask them to consider allowing the vaccinations for the sake of others.

## EXERCISE

In this case study it is possible to focus attention on Diane alone, which is why her beliefs have been explained in detail. What should she do to achieve the highest moral intervention in this case? Before listing options and trying to justify them it is important to note that Diane appears to have some stark choices, and faces a difficult decision.

What do you think? Should Diane:

- Obey the rules as behoves a professional? If you think she should obey these rules against her better judgement, where should a health worker draw the line and disobey? Do you, for instance, think professionals should obey *any* rule that is (explicitly or implicitly) part of their job description? Should they lie? Steal? Coerce? Kill?

- Resign or be sacked? In either case she could be sure that someone else would come along and follow the rules in her stead.

- Somehow manipulate the system to achieve the end she believes to be the most moral, whilst remaining in the job?

## 4.   SPONSORSHIP AND HIDDEN MOTIVES

Professor Ronson is head of a Department of Community Medicine, and would like his department to be involved in as many research projects beneficial to the community as possible. The professor also wishes to employ as many research staff as he can because he well appreciates that it is becoming increasingly difficult for young academics to find worthwhile university posts. He has an idea for a research project to discover the reasons why there is a relatively low use of the medical and health facilities, including a health centre and a well-women's centre, in one part of the city. The area in question is the poorest in the district, and has the highest levels of unemployment and single-parent families, so the uptake rate is predictably low. However, the precise reasons for the under-use of the facilities are not known. Considering that the local population suffers a disproportionately high level of disease and illness it seems unquestionably important to understand more about why the people act as they do.

It is here that the controversy begins. Professor Ronson has exhausted his research budget so he makes it known to potential sponsors and research bodies that he wishes to embark on a two-year project, employing at least one research fellow. Unfortunately for the professor, none of the usual sources of funds wishes or is able to help. However, out

_ continues _

*continued*

of the blue there comes an offer of sponsorship from a famous tobacco company. The company tells Professor Ronson that it hopes to fund worthwhile health research throughout the country and is pleased to say that this is one of its first offers: it is prepared, up to a certain financial limit, to fund for three years a community project of his choosing.

The nature of the problem could hardly be more clear: should Professor Ronson accept sponsorship from a company which trades in a commodity known to cause disease and illness?

*EXERCISE*

Write out the key issues as they occur to you.

State your approval or disapproval of the actions made in this study so far.

Explain what you think Professor Ronson should do. How can he achieve the highest degree of morality in these circumstances?

Explain what you mean by 'the highest degree of morality'.

As far as you can, justify both your theoretical position and your practical proposals.

## 5. TRAGIC CHOICES

Unlike most of these case studies, in which a range of alternatives are possible, this dilemma is at the sharp end of moral philosophy. It sits at the tip of the iceberg, posing the type of predicament[34] typically relished by moral philosophers, where the decision-maker is faced with two choices – both of which she has a *prima facie* duty to make – but can choose only one. Whatever she decides there will be a high price to pay.

The French philosopher Jean-Paul Sartre gave this example of a tragic choice: in the Second World War a young man has to choose between leaving home to fight with the French Resistance, or staying to protect and look after his frail mother, who would have to live alone if he were to leave. What, if he is to be moral, is the young man to do?

There are no more 'tragic choice' case studies in this book because such cases are exceptional. They are simply not the everyday experience of health workers. But occasionally health workers will be faced with them, so it is useful to have some experience of their analysis. However, it is essential to remember that there are no neutral interventions: dramatic ethical dilemmas are merely the most easily seen.

*continues*

_ continued _

## The Nurse Practitioner's Dilemma

Nurse practitioners work from some health centres in the UK and USA. Patients are sometimes able to consult them as an alternative to seeing a doctor. Nurse practitioners can recommend some treatments and will refer patients on where necessary. Many in nursing would like to think the advent of this type of nurse an important step in increasing the status of the profession.

Sandra is a pioneering nurse practitioner who has quickly built up a list of patients who find it easier to deal with her than the doctors. Her clinician partners do not resent this since they recognise the benefits of Sandra's presence, to themselves and the patients.

Sandra is about to attend a seminal national meeting in which a proposal to extend the nurse practitioner programme to all parts of the country will be either agreed or rejected. As an articulate pioneer her attendance is crucial. It could mean the difference between nurse practitioners becoming a recognised part of health services or remaining on the periphery of official health care for the foreseeable future.

As Sandra is about to leave for the meeting the receptionist rushes to tell her that one of her patients is on the phone, threatening to commit suicide and insisting on seeing her. Sandra knows the patient is highly strung and sensitive, and knows too that she is probably the only one who will be able to help. She knows she could very well save the distraught woman's life.

Her dilemma is crystal clear: should she stay to help her patient, or should she go to the meeting to help ensure that more nurse practitioners become available to aid many more people, and possibly save many more lives?

## EXERCISE

Write out the key issues as they occur to you.

Explain which of the options open to Sandra you favour.

Explain why you think your preference would achieve the higher degree of morality. (To stay or to go. Both options might be justified. As you try to justify your choice take careful note of the reasons you give – these are part of your so far unanalysed moral position. Later in the book, once you have the advantage of the Ethical Grid, you will be able to test out the strength of these thoughts.)

# 6. IS COERCION ACCEPTABLE?

Coercion is constraining or compelling a person into thinking or doing something she would not otherwise have done. Is it ever right to coerce a person, either for that person's own good, for the good of society, for human kind as a whole? This question inevitably raises others. For example, is coercion *always* undesirable? Can coercion ever be justified, and if so on what ground? What factors should be taken into consideration before the imposition of a medically defined 'good' on another person? Is it enough that the coercer possesses knowledge impossible or undesirable to transmit to the coerced? Or does another's lack of knowledge place other obligations on the person with superior information?

## The Forthright District Nurse

Anne is a district nurse with strong views against smoking. Her position has become dogmatic over the last six months as a result of her work with two families whose lives have been thrown into temporary chaos by the death from lung cancer of one member of each (in one case the mother and in the other the father). Coincidentally, both deceased used to smoke over 30 cigarettes a day and had done so consistently, for many years. In Anne's opinion there is simply no question that both deaths were directly attributable to their habits. Both people would still be alive, in all probability for 20 or so more years, if they had not smoked.

Anne has now come up with a strategy to deal with smoking problems in other families. She regards smoking as a simple evil which ought to be totally stamped out. She cannot see that smoking has any benefits at all, and nor does she allow any distinction between types of smoker, on any ground. Of course, more sophisticated views than Anne's are possible. For example, one might distinguish between those whose habit harms no one else and those who are smoking in homes shared by young families; or one might distinguish between those smoking who wish to give up and those who believe smoking is helpful to them in some way. Perhaps they are very nervous and smoking helps them relax, and they consider the side-effects of smoking a price worth paying for this relaxation. But Anne accepts no such prevarication. Her aim is to stop the habit, whatever the reasons people have for smoking.

Her strategy has five stages:

Firstly, she always makes it clear that on no account is smoking permitted during her visit to a home.

Secondly, Anne states emphatically that there is absolutely no doubt that smoking causes cancer.

Thirdly, Anne offers, and always leaves anyway, anti-smoking pamphlets and information about why it is stupid to smoke.

Fourthly, Anne deliberately changes her attitude from friendliness to hostility when she knows one of her clients is continuing to smoke despite her advice.

Finally, if her patient continues to refuse to cooperate then Anne's strategy is the severest she can apply. For a time Anne continues to provide the minimum treatment necessary for the condition, but she makes it clear that she could do more, and will – just so long as the patient gives up. If even this fails to produce the desired result Anne refuses treatment until the smoker gives up.

## 7.   DEATH AND THE TRUTH

Jane is an experienced nurse who works on a mixed ward which caters mainly for cancer sufferers at various stages of their treatments. Jane is a Catholic and very single-minded about telling the truth. She believes everybody has a basic right to information about themselves and their circumstances, especially when they are in hospital. And when the relevant information is that they will soon be dead Jane believes she has an absolute duty to tell this to her patients. Not only does she feel obliged to do so, but she argues that certain benefits follow too. Once they know the truth patients are able to prepare themselves, their relatives, and their friends – and to make their peace with God. Jane believes her duty is to impart this information even when a patient is clearly avoiding the issue, even when the relatives ask that the patient not be told, and even if the medical judgement is that the knowledge would cause psychological damage.

Is Jane right in her policy? Is telling the truth the most ethical intervention possible in this type of situation?

## 8.   IS ALL DRUG EDUCATION HEALTH EDUCATION?

Kathy is a thoughtful and conscientious health education officer. Her manager has decided that Kathy will be responsible for the local campaign against 'drug misuse', but Kathy is of the view that some of this material is misleading. Some is quite clearly designed to shock. For example, there are several graphic posters that predict death, physical disability, or a zombie-like existence as an inevitable consequence of using illicit drugs. Furthermore, at least as it appears to Kathy, some of the campaign material sets out to create such myths as cannabis smoking will lead inevitably to smoking or injecting heroin; experimenting with heroin means instant dependency for the user; illegal drugs are the only truly dangerous drugs; all illegal drugs are equally liable to create dependency; and the use of drugs means that the user will eventually be unable to hold down work, or be unable to have a social life with people who do not use drugs. Yet further, the information Kathy has been asked to distribute pays insufficient attention, in her opinion, to the fact that a major cause of dependency arises from addiction to prescribed drugs such as tranquillisers (which can create a dependency from which it is unpleasant and difficult to withdraw).[35]

Kathy hates the thought that a person's major interest in life is finding ways to escape from it. She is strongly in favour of preventing dependency on drugs and of offering alternative means for people to find life worthwhile, yet she is equally earnestly opposed to deception and gross exaggeration of the truth, whatever the motivation of the person who seeks to deceive. Kathy is also increasingly disturbed that, directly and explicitly, she has become an agent for the government. She doesn't think this is necessarily a bad thing but, because she is losing control over what she does, she thinks she has cause for concern.

Kathy has outlined her apprehension to the District Health Education Officer, who referred her to the District Medical Officer, who told her kindly that she must do as she is told by her superiors. This means, in practice, that Kathy is obliged by her employer to ensure that the posters are placed in libraries and other public places, and that Kathy faces a very tricky decision over the content of her lectures to groups of teenagers. She is supposed to follow the official line but knows (she is only 24) that this strategy will be ineffective – even counter-productive with such groups, many of whom will have tried, and if not will almost certainly know people who have tried, illegal drugs and not experienced the tales of horror she has been told to frighten them with. She also has to deal with a similar problem – which she sees ultimately as a question of personal integrity – as she decides on the content of a talk to a group of parents, many of whom will expect to have the government hyperbole confirmed.

*EXERCISE*

Write out the key issues as they occur to you.

Explain how Kathy might act in order to create the highest degree of morality, and offer the strongest defence of this policy that you can.

## 9.   RATIONING HEALTH SERVICES

It's just after midnight. The doors of the Accident and Emergency Department burst open as a semi-conscious man is dragged through by two supporters. One of them half collapses into a chair, hauling his burden with him. The other approaches the reception desk.

'Arapeta's crook, eh?'

'Pardon?' inquires the receptionist. 'What did you say?'

'My bro man, he's shot. We've been on the piss eh, but he can take it man. He don't usually get like this, eh.'

The receptionist looks across the room. She sees an obviously overweight man, in his late thirties or thereabouts, of Pacific Island descent, with swollen features, having difficulty breathing.

'How long has Arapeta been this way?'

'He's not been good for a while eh, a few months, eh bro?' he inquires of the other helper, who nods.

'I think he should see the triage nurse straight away, will you wait just a minute?'

The nurse arrives, briefly examines the patient, calls the doctor, and Arapeta is wheeled away from the reception area.

Two days later, after numerous tests, Arapeta is told he has advanced renal failure, in addition to his diabetes. He needs a transplant and in the meantime could benefit from dialysis, but unfortunately this service is not presently available.

What Arapeta and his friends do not know is that the consultants, managers and hospital lawyers have been involved in hot debate about whether or not to dialyse. The majority verdict was that dialysis should not be offered (though a unit is available) because resources are limited, and it is very likely that more 'deserving candidates' will soon present.

The problem is that Arapeta is not a social asset (at least he is not as most of the decision-makers see it). He is already a diabetic, he has not had a job for years, drinks heavily and has no dependants. To treat him would, at least as one of the consultants put it, 'be an irresponsible waste of taxpayer's money'.

Without treatment Arapeta will die, and his friends are duly informed.

## EXERCISE

Write out the key issues as they occur to you. If you need, you may add any further information necessary to allow a full deliberation. (Is there an explicit policy on dialysis? Has the public been involved? Do coloured people receive dialysis on an equal basis with whites? Do a greater proportion of coloured people need dialysis?)

What are the central moral considerations in this situation?

_continues_

_ continued _____

Do you think the decision-makers' choice has achieved the highest degree of morality?

What could be done differently? What else should be done?

As far as you can, offer a justification and defence of your views.

## 10.  MENTAL ILLNESS

It was a beautiful blue midwinter's day, so radiantly sunny it was hard for Brian Wilson to imagine how anyone could be depressed during it. Yet as a senior psychiatrist in an overstretched and underfunded health service he was ruefully aware that even the most glorious day has only fleeting remedial power.

Dr Wilson parked outside a sparkling white villa, walked briskly through a tidy front garden, and knocked on the stained glass door. It was opened by a tall woman, in her mid-thirties, dressed in a white singlet and shorts.

'Come in Brian, please.' She turned quickly and walked along the hall, her long blonde hair flashing in shafts of sunlight.

'How is he Sarah?' She stopped, and looked straight at him.

'You'll see for yourself in a minute, but it's got worse now. They're trying to get rid of him.'

'Who are?'

'His partners. They sent him a letter today telling him he's in breach of contract. They want him to pack his bags within two days. I've been on to Ken and he's going to look into it for me. Can they do this do you think?'

Wilson had known Paul and Sarah for several years, mostly personally but now professionally, and guessed immediately what had happened. Paul was a GP. A couple of years previously he went into partnership with three others in a local practice, and had been doing well. About nine months ago Paul had become withdrawn and rather depressed, and for the last few weeks had experienced strange thoughts and had been behaving increasingly oddly.

Two weeks ago, with uncanny bad luck, a snatch of his behaviour was caught on film and received national TV exposure for several days. A new casino had just opened, and for some reason Paul went to the opening ceremony (a lavish event, closed to the general public). He interrupted proceedings with shouts and screams: 'parasites', 'leeches', 'capitalist dogs', 'this is sin – all are sinners' and other slogans, more colourful still. The footage was shown every time 'protestors to the Casino' were mentioned on the news, though in truth Paul was the only 'activist' there. It was gruesome publicity for the GP partnership, and had obviously prompted Paul's colleagues to move to banish him.

How nice of them. Just what you'd expect from a caring profession, thought Brian, as he entered the comfortable living room. Paul was sitting in an easy chair, his chin on his chest in unwanted sleep.

'Paul, Paul, how are you?'

Paul shook himself, and with difficulty raised his head and opened his eyes.

'I'm OK. Just tired. This stuff is knocking me out.'

_____ continues _

_continued_

'I think we should change the medication, would that be all right?'

'Yes, sure. I've got to make calls you know.'

'What calls, Paul? Ones to your practice? That letter's bad news mate. Can I do anything?'

'You know Sarah's pregnant again don't you?' Wilson did know. In fact he was as concerned for Sarah and the other three kids as he was for Paul. Sarah was superficially collected, and the pleasant house and uplifting weather imbued the situation with misleading optimism. But when she mentioned the letter her stress had been obvious. She badly needed respite from this mess.

Paul continued. 'Oh yes. That's no problem. Its time I sacked _them_. I have to arrange the concert you see.'

'I thought you were to have the concert last week', Dr Wilson said.

'Oh, yeah, but Kiri couldn't make it. She called and apologised. I said it was OK – sure I can call on a lot of help from around the globe – but I want you Kiri. You owe it to New Zealand.'

'So the concert is still on then?'

'Of course, we're going to have it when we have the regatta down the hill. Michael and Macca are cool about it.'

'Paul, you know there isn't any concert. You know there isn't. Don't go on about it again, please', Sarah said firmly.

'No. OK. I know it didn't work out but I mean I have influence and it will be good. I know it will be good.'

Now Brian changed the subject. 'What were you doing at the Casino?'

Paul laughed. 'Ha, I shouldn't have gone there should I? Not a good scene.'

An image of Paul, kicking, yelling and holding fiercely onto the side of a descending escalator while burly bouncers tried to lever him off it, hung in the doctor's mind.

'No. It wasn't. I'm going to call TV Ten and tell them not to run the clip anymore. OK?'

Sarah said, 'That would be great if you could Brian.'

'And in the meantime', Wilson had more gravity now, 'What do you think about being admitted for a few days? I want to get the meds right, and you need the rest, don't you?'

'What about the concert?'

'There isn't really a concert Paul. It's a grandiose idea, you know.'

'Yes . . . No, I have arranged it and I can't cancel it now. I can't just call Michael Jackson and Paul McCartney and cancel out of the blue . . .'

'You've spoken to them before?'

'Yes. Mostly it is the agent I deal with but don't underestimate what I can do . . .' Paul stopped quite suddenly, and went to sleep again.

'Sarah, we need to get this sorted out. Do you want me to get him a bed?'

'He doesn't want to go to hospital. Does he have to?'

'He may have to, but it would be better if you got him to agree.'

EXERCISE

As far as you can, list the main issues as they occur to you.
Dr Wilson has at least four options available:

1. To do nothing further
2. To change Paul's medication and continue to monitor him at home
3. To persuade him to admit himself to a psychiatric hospital
4. To admit him, without his agreement, to a psychiatric hospital

Which of these options do you think will create the highest degree of morality in this difficult situation?

Can you suggest an alternative policy or policies that would create the highest degree of morality?

Try to justify your opinions and proposals.

## II. DOCTORS AND NURSES

Mary has been a nurse for 27 years, and knows how to handle herself in tense circumstances. This time though, she is not sure how to act for the best.

For the last few weeks she has noticed that Dr Jones, a doctor just into his thirties, has been giving unusually high doses of morphine and other painkillers to terminally ill geriatric patients. From what she knows of him she doesn't believe he is doing anything sinister – she doesn't think he is intending to kill them – but neither does she think he is acting in their best interests. In Mary's opinion the old people are oversedated. They spend their days asleep or sitting by themselves communicating little, if at all. And this, she thinks, is pointless.

Mary spoke to Dr Jones about the dosages, but the conversation didn't go well. The doctor was instantly defensive, and let Mary know right away that 'it is none of your business, OK?' Despite her experience, she was riled at this, and told him straight that it was, and that he ought to think very carefully about what he was doing. Dr Jones interpreted this as a threat (which it was, partly), said he wasn't going to stand for that, and told Mary to get out of 'his ward'. Angry and upset, Mary left.

And now she doesn't know what to do.

EXERCISE

Describe the key issues in this case. What are the main ethical pressures, do you think?

How can Mary act so as to achieve the highest degree of morality?

Why does your suggestion achieve the highest degree of morality?

## 12.   HEALTH IN A BOTTLE?

For six months Pharmaceutical Industries Ltd (PIL) has been providing a legally registered but unsubsidised drug (EAZE) free of charge to 100 chronically ill patients. Most are young – below 30 – and all suffer from a degenerative and incurable lung disorder. EAZE is designed to relieve pain and breathlessness, has done so significantly in 34 cases, moderately in 27, and has had no effect in the rest. Some of the most fortunate group feel so much better that they have returned to work.

This week PIL has written to each patient's doctor to inform them that EAZE is no longer to be offered compassionately. The physicians have called a patients' meeting, which is now underway.

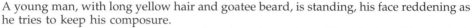

A young man, with long yellow hair and goatee beard, is standing, his face reddening as he tries to keep his composure.

'How can they do this to us? This drug has changed my life. I had nothing to look forward to but now I can drive and I've got a part-time job at the college. If they take EAZE away I'll lose it – shit, I'll lose it all.'

There is a buzz of approval from the others, and claps from some.

'Richard', one of the doctors replies, from behind the table on the stage, 'We've been through this a hundred times. You knew the score when you agreed to this trial. You knew you could have the drug free for six months and that it would stop then. You agreed to it on those terms. It was quite explicit.'

'We knew it, sure we knew it,' a painfully frail young woman stands now, in agitation. 'But we didn't think they'd be such bastards.'

Whoops from her friends.

'We thought they wanted to help us. And we thought – this is going to work and when it does something will change and someone will help us. Hey, we pay taxes so we're entitled anyway. And PIL calls it compassionate supply. We thought they meant it. The drugs haven't run out have they, so where's their compassion gone?'

There's fulsome applause at this.

'We don't make PIL's policy', says the doctors' Chair. 'Like you, we had hoped they would extend the supply particularly because it has worked well for some of you, but they won't have it. If you want to keep on with EAZE it's going to cost you the best part of twenty thousand a year, unless the government agrees to subsidise it, but they say they won't.

'I called William Booth today – the junior Minister. He told me, in no uncertain terms, that the government's drug budget is not a bottomless pit, EAZE isn't a cure, it's expensive, and he isn't going to be blackmailed by the pharmaceutical industry.'

'What do you mean? PIL's been good to us. They didn't have to supply it free at all.'

'He means that PIL has used you first as a trial – to see if EAZE helps people like you – and second as a lobby group: you want EAZE and you could get it if the government chose to help pay for it, so you will put pressure on the Ministry of Health to subsidise EAZE – you're bound to.'

The yellow-haired man pulls himself to his feet again.

'Whose fault is it then? Is it our fault for wanting to get better? Sure, it must be. Is it PIL's fault – they're a business so they have to make a profit, but haven't they given us false hope? And isn't that cruel? Is it the government? They have to ration medicine, we know that, but why this one? I could accept it if I knew they'd looked as carefully at everything else they spend on, but they haven't, of course they haven't.

'Where does this leave us? What am I supposed to do now? Isn't my life worth anything to anyone?'

Distinguish the main components of this complicated case. What are the central moral concerns, as far as you can tell from the information available? Who is behaving well and who is behaving badly? Who is responsible for the health of the volunteers?

Now imagine you are the GP of four of the patients. Assuming you want to achieve the highest degree of morality in this situation, what are you going to do?

## 13.    BUSINESSPERSON OR CARE-GIVER?

Dr Smith has just finished a fraught call to his bank manager. The mortgage rate is up again and the doctor cannot afford the repayments on his new house. As he switches his 'phone off a patient enters, and a perfectly normal consultation ensues.

It turns out the patient has a mild respiratory infection, for which the GP prescribes a broad spectrum antibiotic. He is 98% sure it will do the trick, but he asks the patient to come back to see him in four days time, so he can be certain the antibiotic is appropriate.

This, one might think, is normal and proper practice. But there is a difficulty. Dr Smith works in a country where people of reasonable means (like his patient) have to pay a fee each time they consult. This means, of course, that it is in the doctor's personal interest that the patient makes a follow-up appointment.

Clarify the main points at issue in this case.

Assume that Dr Smith genuinely wants to work first and foremost for the health of his patient. Given this, did his intervention bring about the highest degree of morality or not? Explain your reasoning.

## 14.   WHAT SHOULD THE LECTURER DO?

The second-year medical students have written a petition and all 121 of them have signed it. The petition asks the Dean of the Medical School and the Vice-Chancellor of the University to act immediately to reform the medical school curriculum. Here is part of it:

We the undersigned petition that medical students are given the same standard of education – with the same level of intellectual challenge – as all other students of this University. Though facts and skills are essential to us as future doctors we entreat:

   a. that the first-year programme be altered so that students do not repeat material already studied in school
   b. that pre-clinical teaching staff coordinate to ensure that material is not repeated
   c. that a distinction is made between essential, recommended and optional learning (we presently have to spend days cramming factual material we will never use, which will soon date, or which can be easily looked up if we need it)
   d. that the ethics, sociology, psychology, humanities and communication components be increased as the pre-clinical load is reduced
   e. that time for student directed learning be increased substantially . . .

Dr Crossley, a young ethics lecturer, has repeatedly encouraged and supported the students in these views, and is delighted that they have written the petition. However, when the second-year rep. asks him to sign it, he is not sure he should. Crossley is approaching the end of a three-year fixed term contract, has made both friends and enemies at the Medical School, and is learning that job security comes at a price. If he signs it the Dean will notice – and the Dean is shortly also to rule on whether Crossley's contract should be extended or the job advertised anew.

*EXERCISE*

Clarify the main points at issue.

Is this a health issue?

Should Crossley sign the petition?

How can Crossley best achieve the highest degree of morality?

Explain what the lecturer should do, and why he should do it.

## 15. A RIGHT TO HEALTH CARE?

Dr Walker is quietly explaining to a chronically ill elderly patient that she is not going to recommend further heart surgery. An auxiliary overhears the conversation and anonymously informs the patient's son – Donald Spencer – a prominent lawyer.

Spencer makes inquiries and discovers that though the operation is risky in a woman of 81 it is clinically indicated and – if successful – could increase her mobility and extend her life. He tells his mother what has happened and what he is going to do. At this she begins to cry. She tells him that Dr Walker is a lovely woman and she doesn't want to cause her any trouble. She also says that she is not afraid to die and she hopes a younger person will benefit from the operation instead.

Donald is furious. He tells his mother that he hears the doctor speaking, not his Mum. Dad would never forgive you if you give up now. You are being discriminated against on the ground of age. This is a human rights issue and I'm going to fight tooth and claw to get what you are entitled to. His mother merely sighs, and sinks back on her pillow.

Her son walks purposefully from the room, in search of Dr Walker.

### *EXERCISE*

As with all the exercises, add further information if you need it.

Imagine you are either Dr Walker or Donald Spencer. What are the key issues from your point of view? Why are these the most important issues? Is this basically a human rights issue as Spencer thinks, or are there more important moral considerations?

How should Walker respond to Spencer's angry request to operate on his mother? At this crucial point, how should Dr Walker bring about the highest degree of morality?

## CONCLUSION

This chapter has offered fifteen studies of the sorts of situations which may be faced by health workers. It is hoped that the chapter will serve both as a source of teaching material and as background to the discussion contained in the remainder of this book.

Most of the case studies are not dramatic. Some may have appeared rather ordinary, perhaps even to the point where it was difficult to see how they are to do with ethics at all. But each, when analysed and thought through, raises moral questions of immense significance. All health workers – nurses, doctors, auxiliaries, chaplains, social workers, non-medical staff, consultants, managers, teachers, administrators, and patients – are involved in daily interaction in the moral realm. The secret is to recognise this. Once a health worker is aware of the extent to which morality impregnates her work she can take steps to ensure that she directs her activity towards boosting morality in every situation.

# PART TWO

# The Search for the Truly Moral

# CHAPTER FIVE

# The Search for Morality

## INTRODUCTION

In order to give the best answers to the question 'How can I intervene to the highest moral degree during everyday interventions?' health workers need to understand more about the nature of morality. Consequently, this chapter embarks on a search to discover clear examples of morality. This turns out to be a false hope, but a solid base for ethical practice is unearthed nevertheless.

The problem with the ambition to find 'the truly moral' is that people hold beliefs and values whose truth or falsity cannot be objectively assessed. The statement 'water boils at 100 degrees Celsius at sea level' is testable. It can be shown to be true provided the definitions included in it, and the method of testing, are agreed. But the statement 'it is right to perform euthanasia on a patient who has repeatedly requested it' cannot be tested. It may be possible to establish how many times and under what conditions the patient expressed the wish, but it is impossible to discover experimentally whether or not a health worker would be morally right to assist.

This basic difficulty is further elucidated in this chapter. Afterwards, various attempts to resolve value conflicts are discussed, and five possibilities are considered. These are:

1. Finding some ultimate value or ordering of values.
2. Finding a set of rules.
3. Appealing to the law.
4. Settling for relativism.
5. Making an appeal to the relevant facts.

## THE QUESTION OF VALUE

Any answer one might give to the problems raised in the case studies (Chapter Four) must involve some reference to values. For instance, if you feel that Kathy (the health education officer instructed to carry out a radical campaign against drug misuse) is right in her misgivings, then though your thinking may be based on an assessment of likely consequences, at some point opinion must also have a role. Perhaps it will be thought that Kathy should have more autonomy, or that the public has a right to be informed rather than frightened, or that teenagers should be told the bare truth, or that drug use is not a medical issue. Whatever the case, these are value judgements.

The opposite point of view, for instance that Kathy should conform to the wisdom of her more experienced superiors, or that any course of action is justified if it helps eliminate drug abuse, also rests ultimately on values.

How can such stark value conflicts ever be resolved? This chapter puts forward one answer, but first it is necessary to clarify something of the nature of value.

# WHAT ARE VALUES?

'Value judgements' and 'value-laden statements' are often discussed in moral philosophy and associated disciplines. But what do academics mean by these phrases?

## DIFFERENT SORTS OF VALUE

It seems natural for us to consider some physical things more valuable than others – a motor car, for instance, usually seems more valuable (both financially and practically) than a bar of chocolate. We also tend to think of less tangible things as more or less valuable. Most of us consider that happiness is to be valued above misery, that life is better than death, that pain is bad, that work and creativity are to be admired, that owning property is desirable, that truth-telling is worthwhile, and that trying to help friends is important.

## DISTINGUISHING VALUES

How can different types of value be distinguished from one another? And how can this be done so that more light is thrown upon the nature of morality?

The analysis of values given here is by no means exhaustive. However, it is useful to note (1) that different types of valuing have different ethical implications and (2) that all valuing is done by subjects who exist within a wider culture.

## I.  DIFFERENT TYPES OF VALUING HAVE DIFFERENT ETHICAL IMPLICATIONS

If a person values a principle such as 'the truth must always be told', then her conviction can have implications for ethics in the dramatic, persisting and general senses. However, if a person holds an aesthetic value (if she values a picture or a poem, for instance) or another type of intangible value (perhaps she values a relationship) then the mere fact that she has the value does not necessarily raise dramatic or persisting ethical issues – although maintaining any value always has some bearing on ethics in the general sense (because ethics in the general sense has to do with how a person chooses to live her life, and values are necessary foundations of social behaviour).

## Types of Valuing

The following categories are not impervious, and overlap in significant ways. They are, however, a helpful clarification in the search for morality.

Most simply, a person can be said to have a value when he finds something – anything – valuable. More specifically:

i. It is customary – at least in wealthy societies – for people to value *physical things*, such as compact disc players, money, and pets (either as means, ends or both).

This type of valuing (and all the other types listed below too) can be said to relate to morality in different ways, dependent upon what is meant by morality, and dependent upon which part of the iceberg is perceived as most important at a particular time. Consider your neighbour's house, for example. If morality is merely a question of right and wrong (a form of dramatic ethics) and it is thought that certain moral rules or commandments define what is right, then valuing property will be either right or wrong depending on how you look at the world. If it is a moral rule that it is wrong to covet another person's property, and you covet your neighbour's house, then valuing that physical thing is morally wrong. If the moral rule is that coveting other people's property is good (perhaps because it may inspire greater effort on your part) then valuing that physical thing is morally right. Furthermore, if you value your house and there is *no* ruling about whether *this* is right or wrong, then valuing this physical thing is neither morally right nor wrong, according to the 'right and wrong' view of ethics. (Seen from other parts of the iceberg the question: is it moral to covet my neighbour's house? can look quite different, and is certainly more complex than the 'right and wrong' view allows.)

ii. It is obviously possible to value objects – works of art and beautiful gardens, for instance – for their *aesthetic qualities*. Again, whether or not such valuing has a moral aspect depends upon what morality is said to mean.

iii. Similarly, it is possible to value *intangibles*, such as friendship, introspection, and creativity.

iv. It is possible to value *principles*. Whether or not these should be described as moral principles depends on what they are and – again – on how morality is defined.

If one values moral principles then it becomes necessary to reflect on them, to conceive of them,[1] and to arrive at judgements about whether or not they are worth holding and are consistent with other principles espoused. If a person holds principles that are in some way incoherent then it is her task – as she thinks about how she should live – to make incongruities apparent, so she might improve her personal reasoning. For example, if a person holds the principle 'all life is sacred' and is therefore absolutely opposed to vivisection, yet also believes that in order to protect national sovereignty it is fundamentally right to go to war, then she is not making sense and must decide which principle is most important.

v. It is possible to value *ideologies*, such as patriotism, liberalism, fascism or communism.

## 2.   ALL VALUING IS DONE BY SUBJECTS WITHIN A CULTURE

All human beings capable of intellectual reflection have values. Some of these may be innate (we seem to be biologically programmed to value our own lives and those of our offspring, for instance) but any attempt to give a comprehensive list of 'innate' values would be a ceaselessly controversial exercise.

Some values undoubtedly depend upon the culture and era in which the subject exists. For example, paid work is almost universally valued in contemporary society, but such valuing is possible only if such an institution (work for a fee) exists.[36] Furthermore, given the existence of something potentially valuable, people can obviously be encouraged to value it (this is what advertisers do all the time) – a phenomenon which prompts important questions about the difference between human values and morality. For instance, it is in the interests of capitalist businesses that people value paid work but – just because paid work has become a desired social norm – does this mean it is a moral activity?

### Morality or Value – Which Is Basic?

It is interesting to ask which notion – human value or human morality – is basic?

Options:

i. It is possible that cultural values create all moral principles and reasoning.
    If this were the case morality would depend entirely on human values generated by prevailing cultural norms. Whichever values were predominant in a particular culture would be the source of that culture's moral principles. For example, if 'social stability' and 'racial purity' were fundamental values then – in that culture – moral principles would be specified in such a way as to perpetuate them.
ii. It is possible that cultural values and morality are independent.
    In this case it would be possible, for example, to say with moral authority that although racial purity is valued, polices to ensure it are nevertheless unethical.
iii. It is possible that cultural values and morality are partially separate and partially dependent (which is the proposal advocated in this book).
iv. It is possible that moral reasoning and moral principles create cultural values. (Note though, that if this were the case morality would somehow have to exist beyond or before culture. And one would expect different cultures to have similar basic values.)

## CONSOLIDATION

A link has been established between human value and morality, although the precise nature of this association remains at issue. In the section which follows it is shown that values are an essential part of health work. This, of course, is further evidence of the depth of health work's moral content.

# VALUES PERMEATE ALL HEALTH WORK

It can be tempting to think that work for health is value-free – that some endeavours are good and desired by all. Indeed, it can seem obvious that there can be no question that curing disease, illness and injury is good.

Of course, in many situations – perhaps most – medical care undoubtedly ought to be described as a good thing, but it is not necessarily so. Is it, for example, unequivocally moral to attempt to cure pneumonia in a patient who is suffering the final stages of terminal cancer? Is it moral to perform a hip-replacement operation on a 90 year old suffering from senile dementia? Is it moral to allocate scarce kidney dialysis wholly on the basis of predicted life years? Is it moral to pin the broken leg of a man condemned to be executed the following day?

There are, furthermore, an indefinite number of specific choices that must be made in everyday practice (how many patients should I see each day as a GP? If I don't know something or am unsure, should I admit this to the patient?), there are choices of ward policy in hospitals (should we set a weight and gestation limit below which we will never attempt to resuscitate a neonate?), and there are choices which concern the shape and organisation of health services as a whole (where budgets are limited, which ought to be the priority – heart transplants, cures for acne, or disease prevention campaigns?).

Careful reflection on health care practice will inescapably reveal that all work for health – every last bit of it – is at some point inspired by a human value that has been chosen (implicitly or explicitly) from alternatives. And this, in turn, means that decisions about what a health service should be doing and how it should be organised are not unassailable but rest firmly on the shoulders of those who have the power to change them (a category which includes all health workers, even though most of us have little or no direct influence).

## EVEN ADVICE TO EXERCISE IS NOT VALUE-FREE

Exercise is commonly regarded as an unquestionably good activity, something anyone who is fit enough ought to do. Some people even go so far as to argue that people have a duty to exercise, since by exercising they stand a better chance of avoiding disease and illness that might adversely affect others (family members for example) and place avoidable financial burden on the State.

### A Typical View that Advice to Exercise is Value-neutral

'Everybody knows exercise is, as a matter of fact, good for you. So it must surely be true that well-intentioned advice to exercise sensibly must be a good that everyone will agree about. Advice to exercise, then, is objectively good advice, and as such must be considered value-free.'

But it is not value-free. To think it is is to make the mistake of believing that what you like is what everybody else likes – or at least ought to like 'if only they knew what was good for them' – and to believe that your preference holds true universally. To make this mistake is to underrate the opinions, knowledge, attitudes, and experiences of other people.

The discussion below is not intended to convey the impression that there is no practical or moral difference between exercising conscientiously and smoking 40 cigarettes a day while driving everywhere. Obviously, not all health advice depends solely on subjective value. There are objective elements to much of it (in the above case, the effects of exercise and smoking can be measured). However, even advice to exercise is enigmatic, for the following reasons.

### a)   There Is No Agreed Definition of Fitness

One of the most commonly espoused goals of exercise is 'fitness', yet surprisingly there is no agreed definition of this term. In fact it seems impossible to offer a universal standard of fitness because people have different physiques, are of varying ages and of different sexes. The actual goal for individuals – the personal target they choose to call fitness – will always depend to some extent on subjective opinions about what fitness is, and about what activities they want to be fit for. A decision about whether stamina, suppleness, muscle development, or some combination of these factors is of most importance for personal fitness can be informed by detailed measurement and investigation, but must ultimately depend upon a judgement about which is desirable.

Furthermore, any person's fitness will be influenced to some degree by prevailing social trends (compare, for instance, pictures of Western women in the Victorian era, the 1960s, and the 1990s). The very idea of fitness cannot be entirely separated from fashions in body shape, the sorts of physique needed to enable a person to take part in popular pursuits, and trends in preventive medicine and health education. Thus a statement 'Andy has optimum physical fitness' will rest both on statistical comparison and human definition and social trend.

### b)   Advice to Exercise Can Lead to Undesirable Consequences

Not everybody wants to exercise. Some people find the activity boring, tiring, painful, or just a waste of time. It is not inconceivable that constant advice to exercise might force people into doing something, perhaps trying jogging, against their real wishes. What's more, if people consistently refuse to exercise despite well-meaning pressure, advice to exercise could create guilt, stress and unnecessary anxiety about the damage not exercising could be doing. Moreover, there are significant risks of addiction, injury and even death – associated with exercise.[37] Advice to exercise does not lead to desirable ends in every case.

---

**An illustration of the extent to which values permeate health work interventions: the health visitor, the doting daughter, and the *Sporting Life***

---

Carole, a health visitor in the Handsworth area of Birmingham, UK, cares for an elderly woman called Veronica, who lives with her daughter Maggie. Carole has worked in the area for just over three months. She is 25 and, despite her demanding job, still rather shy and reserved. Carole's parents have lived in Harborne (a prosperous area of Birmingham, markedly different from Handsworth) for 23 years, and Carole has not yet left home. She reads the

*Daily Mail*, always dresses 'smartly and sensibly', and could be classified as 'lower middle class' (both her parents are school teachers). She hopes soon to move from Handsworth to a more rural 'patch'.

Veronica and Maggie live in a Victorian terraced house which has been divided into two flats by their landlord. They have a feud with the couple who occupy the other flat, who (they say) do not keep their three Alsatian dogs quiet enough. Veronica's condition prompted the visit in question, since she had recently had a urinary infection, and her doctor thought it appropriate to keep a friendly eye on her progress.

Veronica is in her mid-seventies and, when Carole arrived, was sitting quietly in her armchair, slim with grey hair tied back in a neat pony tail, with a grace and elegance that sometimes accompanies age borne stoically (*). Maggie the daughter, in blatant contrast, is short (less than 5 feet tall) and very fat indeed, almost comically round, behind huge owl spectacles. She is in her early thirties.

Carole spoke to Veronica, who tried to reply but was repeatedly interrupted by the ebullient Maggie. It was established – eventually – that the urinary infection and sporadic incontinence had greatly improved, and was no longer a worry. Instead, Maggie seemed obsessed with the desire to have her mother fitted with a hearing aid. Maggie's argument was that her mother had difficulty hearing some television programmes, although Carole could see she obviously had no trouble catching what her daughter was saying. Much to Maggie's irritation, Veronica steadfastly refused to try a hearing aid. She said she didn't want to be a nuisance, and anyway she didn't need one. Carole noticed, with regret, that Maggie treated Veronica as if she were a little girl, despite her still impressive manner and appearance (*).

Maggie was unstoppable on the topic of herself and her mother. She explained to Carole, who knew already, that both she and Veronica were dependent on the State for their income (*), and then introduced the six cats, each of which was contemptuously self-satisfied and very well fed (*). Maggie bubbled with news of her mother's recent medical history, and of her own career 'under the doctor' too. She was pleased – even proud – that she was to pay a visit to the surgery that evening. It seemed to Carole that her main motivation was her mother, which was rather a shame because Maggie was undeniably articulate and intelligent(*).

The consultation took place in an unashamedly grimy living room, which had not been cleaned or vacuumed for months. It smelt old-house musty, with a mingling of stale sweat and food. The room was untidy in every imaginable respect and, although only small for a living room, was home to an enormous electric fire, flanked by two equally intimidating television sets.

It was three o'clock in the afternoon. Carole had obviously interrupted Maggie during a meal since she could see, sitting at a dangerous angle atop a cluttered sideboard, a plate stacked high with chips, sausage, baked beans, lamb chops and gravy. Carole could not help thinking that 'a heart attack on a plate' was really the last thing Maggie needed in her obese state (*). And, in Carole's eyes, what was worse was that most of the papers littering the room were recent copies of the *Sporting Life* (*), a paper for horse racing punters. The latest edition lay open on the arm of a big soft chair – obviously Maggie's – placed only 3 feet away from the right-hand television (*). Maggie had been standing for the last few minutes, in which time two of the cats had moved in on the cushions, and another was eyeing the portable trolley by the side of the chair.

Carole looked for an opportunity to leave. She thought she might hasten her departure by offering to take Veronica's pulse. Maggie accepted this proposal on her mother's behalf — on condition that she had her pulse taken as well — at which Carole was mightily relieved that she could at last do something vaguely medical. At least now she could say she had visited the family to further their health, or so she reasoned.

As she left, Carole thought she would be very depressed if she had to live a life like that in conditions like those. At the very least she would have made the effort to redecorate in pastel shades.

## Comment

The above situation is saturated with values and value judgements, some of the most obvious of which are indicated like this (*). There is valuing of relationships (Maggie and Veronica), valuing of aesthetics (the appearance of Veronica, the appearance of the room), valuing of lifestyle (the horse racing hobby), valuing of cleanliness (or not), valuing of personal lifestyle, valuing of health (Carole's understanding of health is different from Maggie's — Carole would *never* eat like that for fear of the morbidities associated with obesity) and valuing of technique (the medical intervention as the pulse was taken). On top of these values there are specific moral judgements — judgements of right and wrong about which the three characters disagree. For instance, Carole is of the opinion that Maggie is morally wrong to treat her mother as she does (Carole also believes Maggie is morally wrong to treat herself as she does), while Maggie has no doubt that she is justified in her actions. And not only are statements such as 'Maggie is a bad daughter' value-laden, but far less overtly judgemental statements such as 'Maggie is overweight', 'Maggie eats unwholesome food' and 'Maggie's house is a mess' also have subjective content.

In the example, many of the value judgements will be reasonably clear to outside observers, though not so apparent to those directly involved. Value judgements such as these do not occur only in the context of professional health work interventions, nor only between people who come from different class backgrounds. On the contrary, value judgements are made in the great majority of human encounters, even those where people share the same values.

It is vital that health workers become more accomplished at recognising the varieties of values that come into play. Much bad feeling, and many disputes over 'moral matters', come about simply because alternative values are not recognised as potentially plausible possibilities (seen through the eyes of someone who conceives of the world differently). Each side tends to regard their own position and outlook as right, and that of the 'opposition' wrong. Yet if the values are spelled out and clarified it becomes far easier to see the situation from other perspectives. (Is Carole totally correct in her view? Is Maggie truly mistaken — isn't she happy? Is she really morally wrong to act as she does? What are her priorities? Are they so unreasonable?) This way it becomes easier to gain a fuller picture of what is going on. It becomes possible to take a different way of thinking seriously and to appreciate why another person values something you do not.

# EVANGELICISM – A FALSE START

Certain people are moral evangelists who attempt to find their way through the proliferation of values in two inadequate ways: by resort to rhetoric rather than reason, and by appeal to a single value, or set of values, as absolutely morally correct. Throughout the ages the moral evangelists' slogan has been 'there is no alternative'.

## AN EXAMPLE

In 1986 there was (in Britain) a well-publicised controversy over the rights of parents to be informed, by general practitioners, if an under-age daughter requests contraception (the legal age for consent to sexual intercourse in the UK is 16). The issue hinged on the question of whether or not parental consent is necessary. Mrs Victoria Gillick, a self-appointed campaigner for parents' rights, wanted to protect the authority of parents over their offspring. Her position – which she said was the only morally tenable one – was that sexual intercourse under the age of consent is unequivocally wrong. From this she went on to insist that anything which encourages it (for instance, the prescription of contraceptives) must be bad, regardless of any other good that might come about (a reduction in teenage pregnancy, for example).

Mrs Gillick gave us a classic example of moral evangelism. However, ethical extremists do not belong exclusively to right-wing political groups or religious persuasions. There are, for example, many left-wingers who are just as dogged. The Labour MP Clare Short once famously introduced a Bill to outlaw the publication of pictures of topless women in newspapers. She argued that such pictures exploit women and encourage male violence. Her argument has merits, in my opinion, but it is not the only morally supportable view, and there is evidence both for and against it.

Moral evangelists picture controversies as stunningly clear-cut. For them, there is always one entirely correct position (their own) while every other option is equally wrong. The moral evangelist understands morality only in the dramatic sense. It is her misfortune to be able to see only the tip of the iceberg. Indeed, the evangelist misses so much it is tempting to conclude that she hardly discerns the moral issues at all.

# CAN VALUE CONFLICTS BE RESOLVED IN A MORE SATISFACTORY WAY?

There are five conceivable routes towards the resolution of value conflict – five paths to consider in the search for the truly moral.

## I.   FINDING SOME ULTIMATE VALUE OR ULTIMATE ORDERING OF VALUES – THE QUEST FOR OBJECTIVE MORALITY

It is commonly believed that some acts are so obviously ethically correct that any sane person must define them as moral.

For example:

- The absolute truth should be told at all times
- Professionals are morally obliged to perform their duties to the best of their ability
- Never do anybody any harm in health care
- At all times the health worker must encourage the maximum possible autonomy in the lives of everyone with whom she deals

It is often further imagined that several such 'ethically correct' statements can be combined to form an objective moral system.

## Analysis

The four statements above are among the most frequently outlined moral principles in medicine and health care. However, by careful analysis, it is possible to show that they are questionable, and that their morally authoritative appearance is deceptive.

There are at least three ways to analyse statements of this sort.

### Way One

*The apparent maxims can be examined individually.* To illustrate with the first: is it certain that a health worker should tell the truth in *all* cases? The answer is hardly clear-cut. Indeed, it is not always obvious what the truth *is*. Which writer on nutrition should the health worker refer to for his advice to the client? Which authority on immunisation should the health carer consult? How probable must a diagnosis be to be described as true? Is the truth about HIV and AIDS the same in 1998 as it was in 1988?[38]

It has been argued that there is a difference between 'telling the whole truth' and 'giving a client a true picture'. Much health work involves specialist knowledge, and Western medicine is based on the study of complicated scientific disciplines. To tell the client 'the whole truth' about a particular condition, to explain the biochemistry, the physiology, and the histories of like conditions in other people, might not be feasible. There may be little time, and a proper understanding might require the client to have considerable prior knowledge. Inevitably, the most pertinent points have to be selected by the health worker. Furthermore, it may be her opinion that the client has been given a 'true picture', but her opinion will not necessarily be shared by a different health worker, even from a similar background.

A related complication concerns the extent to which a health worker should be honest about her true feelings. What if she thinks her patient is obnoxious and idle? To tell the whole truth in these circumstances would mean telling a client her opinion about him, and this is unlikely to be the best way to encourage his recovery.

Further uncertainty can occur if a health worker has factual information which might be detrimental to a client, or that he is holding in confidence. For instance, a health worker might be aware that a client's wife is seeing another man, and knows this is a significant factor in explaining the wife's recent offhand behaviour, which is depressing the husband and causing him to smoke more heavily than usual. In this case the information held by the health worker is both true and relevant to the client's health concern, but should it be conveyed? It seems impossible to argue that it is unambiguously right that it should.

### Way Two

*The maxims can be applied to specific situations to see how they work out.* Consider, for instance, the apparently moral statement: at all times the health worker must encourage the maximum possible autonomy in the lives of everyone with whom he deals.

It is not difficult to imagine real situations in which this expression is, at best, uncertain. Suppose you are introduced by a friend (who knows you are a health professional) to an acquaintance of his who has been taking a range of drugs, now wants to move on to heroin, but is uncertain of the safest way to inject himself. He has read about the drug and its risks and claims he has made an autonomous choice to experiment with it. As a health professional, do you encourage him in his decision (perhaps even injecting the heroin for him) or do you inform the police? If you justify a decision to tell the police by arguing that this will ultimately encourage the drug taker's autonomy in the future (on the ground that if he is prevented from using drugs he will eventually have a wider range of opportunities from which to choose) you will still have acted against the statement in the short term (and a drugs conviction may close more doors than it opens). To give another example, how can the dictum be obeyed by a health worker who knows that a man has a sexually transmitted disease and is taking sexual partners without informing them of his condition? How is this man's freedom to direct his life to be encouraged without decreasing the autonomy of his unsuspecting partners?

### Way Three

A third method of analysis is *to study apparently objectively moral maxims in the light of other ethical theories.* Knowledge of these alternative theories should temper any tendency to make sweeping, unreflective statements. Given a decent understanding of technical ethics, any statement can be assessed from the point of view of any ethical theory, to see whether that particular theory would uphold or reject it. For example, a utilitarian health professional might well take issue with the position that the guiding principle of health work is to harm nobody. A utilitarian might believe that in many cases it is right to harm some people in order to ensure the maximum benefit for the remainder.

## 2.   FINDING A SET OF RULES – THE QUEST FOR A BINDING MORAL CODE

Some people think inquiry in ethics is nothing more than a matter of finding the proper set of moral rules. Their idea is that once the right rules have been uncovered there will be no unresolvable ethical problems. But this point of view is mistaken. Ethics cannot be adequately undertaken merely by following rules.

Throughout history most moral philosophers have held that ethics has a connection with rules and rule-following, but only a few have argued that the ultimate goal is to generate universally applicable rules. Certainly, much ethical inquiry is aimed at the justification of ways of acting that, if well formulated and consistently followed, can guide civilised human conduct, but this is not the complete story. It is an error to expect moral philosophy to come up with a set of statements – some sort of Midas formula – that will always turn a tough dilemma into a golden solution. A more achievable aim of ethical exploration is the clarification of thinking, arguments and problems, the disclosure to decision-makers of the full range of possibilities open to them, and the elucidation of different points of view and ways of reasoning.

The flaw in thinking that ethics is only a question of finding the right rules is that there are no rules capable of providing the best answers to all possible life situations – no moral principles that can be sensibly applied across the spectrum of human experience.

No moral rule exists that cannot be justifiably broken. Take any example of an apparently binding moral rule, and it should not be too difficult to imagine circumstances in which it would be better to transgress it. It is, for instance, widely accepted that it can sometimes be better to lie than tell the truth, and robbing the rich to feed the poor has an established moral pedigree. Even working for health is not a binding rule since a person has to make a commitment to do this, and may decide it is not a path she wants to follow.

Never murder (where murder is defined as the intentional killing of another human being) looks, at first sight, to be a universal rule, but even this dictum can be legitimately ignored in certain circumstances. (Not everyone will agree that murder can be justified of course, but the point is that morally plausible defences of murder can be offered.) Capital punishment (the intentional killing of another human being sanctioned by law) used to be morally acceptable in all European societies, but now is not. However the majority of citizens, when polled, are in favour of it, and are therefore in favour of breaking the moral rule 'never murder' in certain circumstances (a majority is usually found to be in favour of murder in wartime, in self-defence and in defence of property too).[39]

Euthanasia is said to be murder by those opposed to it (and by most legal systems in the developed world), yet is mercy-killing to its advocates. Whatever one labels it, euthanasia is intentional killing that some would allow and others prohibit – and this surely brings the moral status of the dictum 'never murder' into question.

## Rules of Games and Rules in Ethics Are Not Synonymous

In competitive games, such as cricket and soccer, binding rules are essential. Without rules to give structure such games could not exist. The rules of cricket and soccer have been carefully developed in order to cater for every situation that might arise in a game. It is a prerequisite of playing such games that players agree that every rule is legitimate. Then, if they violate any, players must accept whatever punishment is laid down. In competitive games it is usual to have an independent judge whose role is to make sure the rules are followed.

Games are artificial, created by people who have defined the limits of each type of contest. A game is like a world apart. Within it, the rules are absolute and at least while the game is in progress there can be no outside interference with them.

Games are qualitatively different from ordinary life, which is not only vastly more complicated but is not enclosed by unbreakable rules. Of course, human beings create moral rules just as we invent rules for games. However – unlike the rules of rugby or netball – moral rules are usually cast generally, and not spelt out to provide for all foreseeable situations.

Rules are a part of almost all daily behaviour, yet it is important to remember that there are many situations in which rules are not enough. Professional codes of practice are a good example. Codes of practice lay down general principles but cannot advise on their interpretation, explain how to decide between principles which conflict, or indicate when it is best to disregard them and deliberate independently. The following examples taken from codes of ethics show, without the need for any further comment, the extent to which their rules must be interpreted in context:

> Any act or advice which could weaken physical or mental resistance of a human being may be used only in his interest.[40]
>
> A doctor must always bear in mind the obligation of preserving human life.[40]
>
> Members will use appropriately their professional skills in the fulfilment of health education/promotion activities which they believe to be effective.[41]
>
> A doctor must preserve secrecy on all he knows. There are five exceptions to this general principle:
>
> 1. The patient gives consent
> 2. When it is undesirable on medical grounds to seek a patient's consent, but is in the patient's own interest that confidentiality should be broken
> 3. The doctor's overriding duty to society
> 4. For the purposes of medical research, when approved by a local clinical research ethical committee, or in the case of the National Cancer Registry by the chairman of the BMA's Central Ethical Committee or his nominee
> 5. When the information is required by due legal process.[40]
>
> Members will use their professional judgement regarding the confidentiality of information to which they have access, bearing in mind the requirements of the law and the best interests of their clients.[40]

It should be increasingly clear, as this search for morality develops, that health professionals not only need codes of practice (and a certain amount of legal knowledge) but also (and much more importantly) a wide acquaintance with ethical theory and modes of moral reasoning. Given this they can bow to or apply rules where they deem it appropriate, but are also able to apply well-reasoned personal judgement.

The trouble with rules can be summarised like this:

a. If the rules or codes are cast in general terms (for example, 'practitioners should always uphold the highest professional standards') they will either be open to wide interpretation or specific cases will contradict them: where exceptional action is needed morality can be increased by breaking the rules.

b. If the rules are specific it is inevitable that sooner or later cases will occur for which no rules have been laid down.

c. Even if *both* general and specific rules are decreed, problems (a) and (b) persist.

## Rules Should Not Be Ignored in Health Work Ethics

A continuum of positions on rule-following can be pictured. Dogmatically consistent rule-following at one extreme, arbitrary personal choice at the other. Neither of these poles is satisfactory if health work is to achieve the highest degree of morality.

To allow entirely free personal choice by health workers, not guided by rules, is not a workable policy. Health workers need the assurance rules can provide, and health services must operate with consistency if they are to secure public confidence. Furthermore, health workers are legally accountable for their actions, and most are understandably reluctant to do anything without the support of rules. Having said this, it is equally important that no code of practice or set of ethical principles should ever be considered imperative.

## Summary

The *benefits* of having rules and following them are:

a. If rules have been drawn up and agreed then it is likely they will be based upon reasoning and analysis

b. Rules provide useful guides for action

c. Rules will often be public – those who are dealt with by health workers will know at least some of the rules.

The *disadvantages* of always conforming to rules are:

a. People's powers of judgement and decision-making tend to atrophy if not regularly used

b. Whatever the rules, situations will occur where breaking one will produce a higher degree of morality than abiding by it

c. A defining element of moral deliberation is that there must be uncertainty – at least at first. To state beforehand that a particular principle must be upheld whatever the circumstances is to negate morality. Without the possibility of choice moral deliberation is sterile.

## 3.    APPEALING TO THE LAW – THE QUEST FOR MORAL LEGISLATION

## Legality and Morality – a Tangled Web

Legality and morality are not synonymous domains. Professional organisations recommend codes of practice to their members because many types of human conduct are potentially harmful, but do not break any law (being unreliable, being inconsistent, being vindictive, being friendly to some people and arrogant toward others, for instance). Such conduct is arguably unethical, but not illegal.

Lawful behaviours are frequently considered moral, and equally many illegal actions are deemed immoral. However, these are not the only possible classifications. There is a web surrounding this issue which, once untangled, can contribute toward a more complete understanding of what ethics is.

## Clarification by Separation

Note: *laws vary between nations. Unless stated otherwise the laws referred to in this section are based on English law.*

It is possible to make six basic distinctions, all of which may be illustrated with examples. Acts may be judged to be:

### a)   Legal and Moral

There are many examples in this category. For instance, most people agree that it is legal and moral to donate money to charity, to work voluntarily with disabled people, or to listen to another person as he relates his troubles. Indeed some moral actions are legally enforceable, though it is debatable whether actions done under duress can be said to be moral. For example, courts of law compel witnesses to tell the truth as they know it, and most contracts are legally enforceable, which is an official way to ensure people keep promises.

### b)   Legal and Immoral

Morality can conflict with law. The following examples are arguably immoral, yet all are legal. It is necessary to concede the validity of one only in order to recognise the sharpness of the legal/moral distinction.

  i. When a person breaks a marriage vow.
  ii. When a person makes a promise without intending to keep it.
  iii. When a lecturer offers higher grades to a student than his work merits in return for sex.
  iv. When government ministers cut the money available to higher education, and consequently deprive some people of education from which they could otherwise have benefited.
  v. When a soldier kills a person in war.
  vi. When a person is imprisoned purely as punishment, without attempt at education and rehabilitation.
  vii. When governments deprive people of rights enjoyed by others.
  viii. When people, acting under the law, intentionally physically or mentally disable other people. For example, it remains legal in some Arab states to cut off one or both hands of a person found guilty of stealing, and the possession of heroin carries a mandatory death sentence on conviction under Malaysian law.

## c)   Illegal and Immoral

There are many examples of this combination, though in each case it is conceivable that some people will not agree that the acts are immoral. However, it can plausibly be said that burglary, intimidation, violence and reckless driving are both illegal and immoral.

## d)   Illegal and Moral

Like the legal/immoral combination, this category can provoke debate, but it is not unreasonable to suggest that the following actions are both moral and illegal:

  i. When a driver breaks a speed limit in order to take a man suffering from a heart attack to hospital.
 ii. When a group obstructs city traffic by a 'sit-down' demonstration against the use of nuclear weapons.
iii. When a person embezzles money from a wealthy company in order to donate it to children's charities.
 iv. When a charitable organisation breaks a country's import regulations in order to get life-saving food to starving people as quickly as possible.
  v. When a person employed by a Welfare Department interviews a claimant in obvious need, is prevented by a technicality from providing help, and yet falsifies certain of the claimant's details in order that the need can be met.
 vi. When a general practitioner fills out a sickness certificate falsely in order to help her patient. The doctor might, for instance, be unable to find any specific complaint but be of the view that the patient would benefit from time away from work pressures, and so reports a very general condition – stress, depression, or viral illness perhaps.

## e)   Legal and Amoral

With this classification everything depends on the sense of morality invoked. If morality is conceived only in the dramatic sense (ethics at the tip of the iceberg) then most activities will be legal and amoral just because so many of them will not be thought to be in the ethical realm. However, if ethics is interpreted in the general sense – in which all activity has moral import – then few actions can be so described (see the Introduction for expansion of this point).

## f)   Illegal and Amoral

As with the 'legal and amoral' classification everything depends upon the sense of morality in play. For example, if one takes the view that both intentions and consequences must be taken into account, an illegal act done in ignorance can be neither moral nor immoral. For instance, a tourist might park his car illegally in a foreign city without meaning to break any law or even realising he has done anything untoward, and without causing any other person harm. Or a person might genuinely forget to have her car checked for roadworthiness (a legal requirement in many countries) thus breaking the law, but not offending any moral standard (unless the view is taken that law sets the moral standard).

Figure 10 illustrates the six categories.

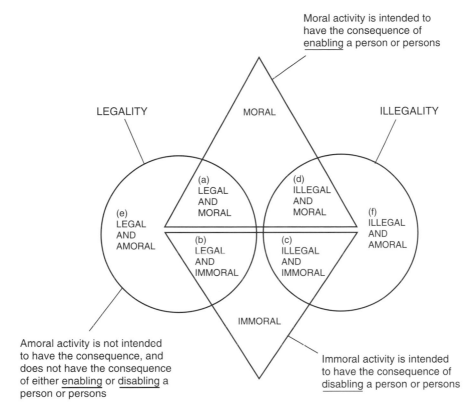

Moral activity is intended to
have the consequence of
enabling a person or persons

LEGALITY   MORAL   ILLEGALITY

(a)
LEGAL
AND
MORAL

(d)
ILLEGAL
AND
MORAL

(e)
LEGAL
AND
AMORAL

(f)
ILLEGAL
AND
AMORAL

(b)
LEGAL
AND
IMMORAL

(c)
ILLEGAL
AND
IMMORAL

IMMORAL

Amoral activity is not intended
to have the consequence, and
does not have the consequence
of either enabling or disabling a
person or persons

Immoral activity is intended
to have the consequence of
disabling a person or persons

**Figure 10**   Distinguishing law and morality

## Summary

It ought now be easy to see that the quest to find the truly moral through legislation is doomed to failure. What is legal and what is moral are not necessarily related. It may be that a system of law is necessary to ensure minimal levels of morality and to maintain social order. But this is not to say that systems of law are therefore always moral systems.

## 4.   SETTLING FOR RELATIVISM – GIVING UP THE QUEST

So far it has been shown that it is not possible to discover a single value that can be said to be objectively moral. Nor is it possible to invent rules or laws guaranteed to produce the most moral outcomes. And thus it might appear that the only solution is to succumb to relativism. But this is an inadequate answer too.

In order to explain relativism it is helpful to contrast it with objectivism.

## Objectivism

There is a metre rule in Paris which sets the standard for any metre length. Objectivists argue that in most walks of life there are standards of truth analogous to the metre rule, even if it is not yet certain what they are. In science, for example, objectivists maintain that researchers are discovering truth about reality, truth about the world as it is independent of human interpretation. In the same vein, objectivists think different sorts of human society can be judged more or less primitive according to how rational they are. This view rests on an assumption that there is an objective standard of rationality to which some of the human race conform. Where societies are found to behave illogically or unreasonably when judged by the standards of anthropologists, objectivists claim these societies are irrational.

## Relativism

Against objectivism, relativists insist there are no objective standards of truth. As far as human society is concerned relativists argue that different social systems operate according to non-universal standards, even though some standards may be held in common. One implication of this is that it is not only morally wrong but conceptually impossible to criticise them on the ground of irrationality. Since some societies operate with different forms of rationality, logic and truth, the anthropologist who assumes to judge an alien culture as 'irrational' or 'illogical' is able to do so only from the standpoint of his own cultural norms, not in line with an objective standard. For the relativist, if society does not conform to the norms the anthropologist calls rational then the other society is irrational only in the opinion of the anthropologist. Societies can be said to be irrational when compared to other societies, but this does not mean that the strange society is truly irrational because there is no external standard by which to judge this. Standards of truth are relative to different contexts.

These opposed positions conflict in moral philosophy too, as the following examples show.

## TYPES OF MORAL RELATIVISM

The following theories are relativist. None refers to an ultimate standard of morality, and each gains strength by denying its existence.

## EMOTIVISM

This point of view was put forward by A. J. Ayer, who believed that the only difference between a statement describing facts and a statement offering a judgement about their morality is the personal opinion of the speaker. For Ayer the statement 'the nurse did not explain the likely side-effect of the treatment' can be distinguished from the statement 'the nurse was wrong not to explain the likely side-effect of the treatment' merely on the ground that the second statement has words added which express disapproval of the nurse's behaviour. This is a value judgement and, according to Ayer, it is not possible for people to contradict each other about statements of value because such statements have nothing to do with truth or falsity. Since everything in the realm of value is a matter of opinion, all one can do is continue to express one's opinions, and continue to give vent to one's emotions.

Furthermore, any apparently meaningful argument about an ethical issue can never be genuine since ethical judgements are kinds of feelings only, based ultimately on the psychological state of each interested individual. All that can be said of each feeling, each emotion, and each value is that each is of exactly equal merit – all opinions are as good or as bad as each other, and since no moral standard exists outside emotion and feeling there is no yardstick against which to measure the differences. Which means, of course, that it is impossible to decide who is right in ethical disputes.

## Where is this Theory Weak?

The trouble with this theory, as with all types of relativism, is that it fails to provide solid ground on which to stand. Not only does it deny the possibility of making moral judgements that can be said conclusively to be better than alternatives, but it implies that to respond according to one's feelings is as desirable as to respond using reason.

Although it is true that value judgements cannot be said to be true or false in the way a statement about the physical world can (just as it is not possible to say decisively that a particular painting or record album is aesthetically good or bad), it is insufficient to say that ethical disputes relate only to people's psychological states. While subjective opinion is an essential part of moral reflection, the real world and the outcomes of decisions taken in it, are an integral part of ethics. To understand ethics properly is to recognise that there is more *at stake* than opinion and emotion: although it is not always possible to reach agreement about values it is often possible to discover which outcomes will most favourably affect those involved.

# EGOTISM

Egotism is more an assertion than a theory, since it equates 'being moral' with the consistent pursuit of self-interest. The moral egotist asserts that what is morally good is what is in his interest: good is what is good for him. Achieving other people's interests is not an equivalent moral good.

Egotism has always been a mainstay of economic theory. The economist's 'rational man' is the self-interested man, the man for whom altruism and respect for others has little or no meaning. The 'rational man' takes other people into account only in so far as they are a threat and in competition for the scarce resources he covets. If morality has any meaning at all for this form of economics it exists only in relation to the desires of individuals.

## Where is this Theory Weak?

One of the difficulties with arguing against relativism is that since he denies the existence of objective standards the relativist has only to state that his version is as good as any alternative. And as far as he is concerned he need not argue further. However, the relativist's opponent should not accept this tactic, but must insist on an examination of the theory's implications, and demand the fullest justifications for its premises. For instance, egotism must depend in some way upon psychology and genetics, which are open to debate and empirical test.

Most health workers will find the egotist account of morality alien since it is diametrically opposed to the values implicit in caring for others. Egotism denies that moral activity is a process of reflection and deliberation which must take account of other people as well as oneself, and as such it is difficult to see how it is a moral theory at all.

## CULTURAL RELATIVISM

For the cultural relativist the question of what is morally right and wrong does not rest finally on the opinions or feelings of individuals. Instead, she believes that moral notions are generated by social arrangements, and that there is no yardstick beyond cultural standards. The ethical codes upheld in one society are not necessarily morally right in another, and it is impossible to decide which view is best. It has, for example, been documented[42] that Eskimos believed it to be morally correct for children to kill their parents while they were still able-bodied, to prevent them becoming senile and decrepit. For most Westerners such behaviour seems clearly immoral: the idea of children putting their parents to death is abhorrent (especially to parents), and remains abhorrent even when the justification for the behaviour is understood. It was apparently an Eskimo belief that people retain the physical bodies possessed at their death in the after-life. Consequently it makes sense to kill people (with or without their consent) in order to ensure they are not disabled in the next world (in my case somewhere around 22 or 23 would have been good). And that is where we must leave matters according to the cultural relativist. Since there is no such thing as objective morality there is no point in trying to arbitrate between the Eskimo and the Westerner.

It is taken for granted by many European citizens that the principles under which we have lived for generations are objectively good. Democracy, free speech, freedom from fear of death at the hand of another, freedom to own property, and equality under the law, are all popularly considered to be fundamentally moral principles. But the cultural relativist begs to differ. She points out that Europeans have not always held such values and may not hold them in the future. Furthermore, there are always some people who would change them because *they* do not regard them as the most moral possible. European morality is objective only in the sense that the majority of the people silently assent to it.

To different degrees, all types of relativism make the claim that the search for morality – at least for an external objective morality – is misguided. Paradoxically relativist theories can provoke the search for universal standards since they tend to inspire the inquirer to give reasons why a practice is morally better than another. Unless this is possible, unless some answer can be found to relativist scepticism, there is no difference between the statement 'you must not kill me because it would be immoral' and the statement 'you must not kill me because I don't want you to'. But there should be the world of difference between them. The first implies that to kill a human being is wrong because it offends against an important moral standard, while the second asserts that it is wrong to kill a human being only because he is interested in self-preservation.

We have an indefinite range of interests that are frequently in conflict. What is needed is some set of standards to provide some arbitration – some sort of moral guidance – in cases where interests are in competition. Fortunately, there is a plausible answer to the relativist. It lies in an appeal to the facts.

## 5.   AN APPEAL TO THE FACTS – THE FOCUS ON WHAT IS

Before a path towards a more solid morality is mapped out it is necessary to elaborate on an important distinction, the difference between what is and what ought to be the case.

### The Distinction Between Ought and Is

This distinction is introduced as a preliminary stage in an argument to pin down the source of morality (at least in respect to health work). The distinction shows that the very idea of morality is partly created by human beings. However, this does not imply that morality has no independent basis.

As we have seen, statements about morality are qualitatively different from statements of fact in that they can never be proven. Armed with this knowledge, it is possible to avoid the trap of thinking that evidence of what *is* is evidence of what *ought* to be.

Consider the following statements:

Eric took $10 from his grandfather's wallet.

Ian took the gun and shot John three times between the eyes.

David donated $50 to Save the Children.

Anne told a lie in order to spare her boyfriend's feelings.

Although it looks as if each statement has intrinsic moral substance, the is/ought distinction shows that the moral content is added by human beings. Without our opinions, impressions and judgements, each statement is nothing more than a factual report (so long as each statement is true). If we assume Eric was stealing, we might think he was morally wrong to take $10 from his grandfather's wallet. But nowhere in the act itself, or in the statement reporting the act, is it possible to discover rightness or wrongness, an 'ought' or an 'ought not'. The bare fact is that Eric removed money from a wallet. He might have been fetching it for his grandfather, or borrowing it with permission, and even if he was stealing it the notion that 'stealing is bad' is a social judgement, not a natural fact.

What is just is, and it is not possible to argue validly from factual premises to moral conclusions. Whenever this is attempted the moral element is smuggled in like this:

Ian took the gun and shot John three times between the eyes.

*Killing people is morally wrong.*

Therefore Ian was wrong to shoot John three times between the eyes.

The first premise is factual, the second (in italics) is not.

## How Does this Help Inquiry into the Ethics of Health?

It is important in the following ways. Firstly, it reinforces the point that there is no objective morality to be discovered in the sense that Mount Everest exists to be discovered. We cannot embark on experimental field trips to find out what is truly right – rather we must use reason. Secondly, the is/ought distinction can make us wary of arguing that because the group of human beings of which *we* are a part acts in a certain way (because the group is as it is) this is the most moral way to behave. Thirdly, and most important of all, we can now begin to understand that although moral judgement has an essentially subjective component, this does not mean it is impossible to base moral principles on objective evidence. Although it is logically incorrect to derive an 'ought' from an 'is', it is not invalid to found a moral theory on matters of fact.

Let us see how this can be so. The moral quality of actions depends at least in part upon the value of what they bring about. In order to know whether some action is morally good it is therefore necessary to understand what is worthwhile in two factual senses:

i. It is necessary to understand what the people you will affect with your actions value (their values are subjective but *that* they value as they do is a fact).
ii. It is necessary to understand that people do not have infinite potential, though they can develop in a wide range of ways. Some of these ways (continuing to breathe, not being in excruciating pain, being able to think) are absolutely necessary if they are to develop at all further. And some other ways (not being injured, not being seriously ill, not being ignorant) are necessary if their further development is to be fulfilling.

Moral actions must intend to promote what is good in one or both of these senses, though how to do this specifically for the best must be the subject of careful deliberation in each case.

Work for health is a fundamentally moral endeavour because it encourages both biological and chosen human potential. Work for health is work to enable in both factual senses (see Seedhouse[5,10] for detailed discussion of these points. Note in particular that the above distinction forms the basis of the 'autonomy flip' in Seedhouse[10]. Point (ii) roughly has to do with *creating autonomy*, while point (i) is concerned with *respecting it*).

This insight undermines the is/ought objection. Being human and possessing a range of worthwhile potentials is a fact which contains an ought. That is, the statement 'Fred is a human being' contains within itself the statement 'Fred ought to be a human being'. This cannot be denied without absurdity.

The precise moral importance of being human is less clear. This book contends that work for health makes the reasons it is valuable to be human explicit, and that those who decide to work for health make a basic moral commitment – uniting the ideas of health and morality.

This argument cannot be made quickly or easily, and has now been developed over several works; however further support must be provided at this point. If it is true that morality cannot be discovered as Mount Everest can, and if it is true that there is no morality beyond human value and thought, morality must lie in what is of central importance to human beings, what human beings have in common – what human beings are for.

# A SEARCH FOR IMMORALITY

## DISCOVERING THE NATURE OF MORALITY BY FOCUSING ON ITS OPPOSITE: IMMORALITY

Because there is a baffling variety of candidates for the title 'truly moral' and no uncontroversial criteria for judging between them, it is sensible to attempt to identify *immoral* actions in order to cast new light on their apparently polar opposite – the moral.

## AN EXAMPLE FROM SOCIAL WORK

This strategy is common in social work, where there is often divergence of opinion about what constitutes a 'good parent'. Does a good parent leave his child in the care of others for long periods? Is the person who has little feeling for her child yet still provides diligently for all material necessities a good parent? Or does a good parent love her child so deeply that she will never let him out of her sight? It is hard to say which parent comes closest to 'the ideally good parent' because this label is so obviously contestable. However, what is important so far as this inquiry is concerned is that although there is endless controversy about the definition of 'good parent', it seems possible to reach universal (or almost universal) agreement about what a bad parent is. For example, it would be very difficult to find a social worker who does not agree that a person who consistently and deliberately inflicts physical and mental harm upon her child, who never considers what might be good for him, and does not intend to produce long-term good either, is a bad parent.

## ON THE OBJECTIVELY IMMORAL: GRAND THIAM

The following hypothetical society is described for two reasons: to give a clear example of immorality and to draw attention to an association between the ideas of health and liberty. If this illustration is thought too fanciful it will be rendered relevant by relating it to real families, familiar relationships, politics and behaviours in the workplace, or to societies unable or unwilling to provide fulfilling work for many of their people.

## THE WAY OF THINGS IN GRAND THIAM

Grand Thiam is a human civilisation which has either existed in the past or will exist in the future – it does not matter which. Despite enviable material wealth its residents are becoming vociferous: demanding power, demanding greater liberty, and demanding the right to decide their own destinies.

This pressure for change is a serious threat to the government's priorities. Grand Thiam is ruled by 100 Elders not allowed to marry or procreate, but who can select their successors without public consultation. For them the ideal society has strong social cohesion, every citizen knows his place in it, there is unquestioning obedience to the law, all industry is able to achieve maximum productivity, and disease is kept to a minimum. They prefer these values over such alternatives as free and uncensored speech, public participation in decision-making, and equal opportunity of access to political power. From the Elders' point of view, the more such values proliferate the more the status quo is threatened.

Through a recently developed cocktail of genetic and educational manipulation the Elders now have the power to engineer their perfect world.

### Dwarfing

Time has moved on and the Elders have used the technology. The 'educational' part of the process made use of a Platonic 'noble lie'. All history books were destroyed and replaced by texts which indoctrinated the belief that a caste system is the only possible pattern on which an orderly society can be based. This propaganda was reinforced by genetic engineering – the insertion of the donkey's 'subservience' gene into human embryos – and the addition of chemicals to the water supply, intended to alter mental states and attitudes. In the early years the plan was effected by weakening the population's curiosity, logical power, and questioning abilities through 'immunisa-tions' universally administered, and by radically increasing the banality of television programmes and newspapers. As the population who had experienced relatively unfettered thought died off the manipulations were stepped up, so all new citizens could be physically and intellectually fitted from birth for their allotted roles (which were defined by various subcommittees of a working party of the Elders' steering group). This not only meant that people's intellectual powers were reduced and clouded, but also that the physiques of some were artificially restricted. The Elders' aim was to ensure the creation and perpetuation of their 'ideal state' through restraining the very existences of the human beings who constitute it.

It was necessary to interfere with the physical development of some children in order to suit them physically for the tasks they were to take on in 'adult' life. This meant that for some jobs, such as the non-automated inspection of pipelines, the cleaning of tower blocks and skyscrapers, and some types of mining, the physical development of some children was halted before puberty, and their intellectual development regulated according to the complexity of the task they were to perform. (If this seems incredible it is salutary to remember the not uncommon practice in India for desperate parents to cripple and mutilate their offspring in order to enable them to beg more successfully.) Many of Grand Thiam's children were intentionally prevented from fulfilling their natural physical and mental potentials in the interest of the society as a whole, as this interest was perceived by the Elders. In other words, these children were deliberately dwarfed.

## A MAJOR CONNECTION: HEALTH WORK IS WORK AGAINST DWARFING

There is something intuitively disgraceful about the process of dwarfing.

Analysis of the theory and practice of health work shows that its underlying sense is the concern to remove or prevent obstacles to physical and mental growth. Health work strives to enable people to bring to fruition the range of potentials that lie latent within them. By educating, by curing disease, by mending broken bones, by developing personal power to conceive – to picture one's situation and future possibilities more clearly – health work is the antithesis of dwarfing.

Since it is an exact counter-balance to dwarfing (or 'the immoral') it follows that the health work endeavour is as objectively moral as it is possible to be. But because there are different types of health work, different senses of moral, and an indefinite range of contexts and ways in which health work can be carried out, it is not possible to say definitely that a particular intervention is *ideally* moral. It is also a mistake to assume that each attempt to create health will be as moral as any other. As was shown in the two situations involving the young footballer with a broken wrist there are degrees to which the enabling (or anti-dwarfing) can be carried out. However, if the intent of the health worker is to enable the enhancing potentials of the person she is working with, if the path she pursues is one which she can justify with integrity, then the work will inevitably be moral.

In the ailing paradigm there is a massive imbalance between the attention given to the physical and all other aspects of people's lives – even though it should be quite clear that the subject matter of genuine work for health is not just bodies but whole people and the external factors which make up their lives. Work for health should be the comprehensive construction and maintenance of the foundations on which people can achieve. In the new paradigm no bona fide health worker will seriously take the view that the end point of health work is nothing more than a non-diseased body. It will be a commonplace that health work does not strive to keep people alive as an end in itself – it does not work only on bodies and treat people as objects. Instead, it will be recognised that a body is given therapy in order to allow the person to go on making real as much of his fulfilling potential as possible.

Work for health can properly be so much more than medical and hospital care and traditional health education – yet the old paradigm is stubborn and hard to shift. It is easy enough to explain this inertia, but very much harder to do anything about it. For example, it is presently uncontroversial that children's eyes should be checked at an early age. The only debate is about how early this should be. Many health authorities recommend that children should have had their eyes examined by the age of three and a half, though some specialists argue that even this could be too late to remedy certain defects.

Defects of vision can be detected and something practical can often be done with immediate effect. This is what the old paradigm is good at. Yet there is in principle no reason why a person whose intellect has stagnated at 36 as a result of a tedious job and unchallenging existence should not be equally a target for a health intervention. A person's intellect is just as much a part of him as his eyes, and its flourishing is arguably even more important if he is to become a mature and interested person. The problem with health work is that the values, political judgement, and empirical evidence involved with intervening with intellectual development are far more obvious, and the options more contentious, than with work with eyes and other physical features. But though this may be a *difficulty* it does not mean that such work is not genuinely part of the endeavour to create more health. In many medical consultations, in conversations between nurses and patients, in some types of health education, in women's health groups and neighbourhood schemes this endeavour is already going on. The extra needed to bring about the best version of the new paradigm is for the health service to acknowledge explicitly the breadth of health work, and to make clear the inescapable conclusion that work for health – within certain legal and moral limits – is work to liberate the fullest possible spectrum of human potential.

## An Objection

It might be argued that although the above account gives a credible view of health, it misunderstands the nature of potential. Because human bodies develop throughout life there are always biological potentials that can be enabled. But this is not so clear in the case of intellectual potentials. It might, for instance, be argued that schooling stops at sixteen because only a minority of people have the potential for higher education, just as only a small minority of people can become athletes or cricketers.

Against this it can be said that the assumption that only physical potentials continue to develop throughout life is based on poor evidence. Work in psychology, psychiatry and education clearly shows the range of intellectual potentials that can be enabled. And there is considerable further evidence that development in logic and reasoning can be impeded (or dwarfed) through lack of practice, lack of expertise, and lack of information.

In short, the problem is this: we have, in developed countries at least, no difficulty in accepting that a working-class child's broken leg should be set so that it will develop well, as it would have if it had not been injured. It is also self-evident that physical obstacles of this sort are not dealt with for only their own sake – only because they are injured, painful or abnormal. They are, of course, tackled in order to restore normal biological functioning, but are also dealt with so that a person can go on to live a fulfilled existence. People are not put back on their feet just for the sake of it, but in order that they can do more and be more satisfied. Physical potentials are enabled in order that further enhancing physical and mental potentials will be liberated as well.[1]

However, although the logic is identical, it is apparently more difficult to accept (1) that the intellect of the child with the broken leg should be encouraged to develop as it would have given the educational opportunities at home and school that more privileged children have, or (2) that the child's emotional development should be brought to the level it could have been were it not for the disabling effect of his parents' broken marriage, or (3) that the child's ability and opportunity to choose throughout life should be encouraged to flourish as fully as possible. But genuine work for health is work directed against the intentional or accidental dwarfing of people. And since every aspect of a person's being is potentially dwarfable, work for health should be correspondingly comprehensive.

## SUMMARY

A number of possible paths towards the discovery of the truly moral have been discussed and rejected in this chapter. What remains is the knowledge that it is necessary to consider human nature and potential empirically, in order to better understand what human beings are for, and so to learn how we should behave toward each other. Although it is impossible to give an objective list of enhancing potentials, and not possible to define what is truly moral, it is possible to be clear about what is immoral. This and the implicit notion of dwarfing are vital clues.

The following points have become clear:

1. There is no morality independent of human beings. What would such a morality be like? The claims of some religious groups that ethical rules have been established by a supernatural entity are opinion only and cannot be tested. If one believes that a deity creates morality then everything is evidence for this, yet if one chooses to disbelieve the claim then nothing counts as evidence for it. Crucially, since there is no evidence that would sway a neutral, the view cannot be empirically sustained. Surely the only possible place to search for morality is in the human race itself.
2. Any opinion of any human being about what is moral and what is not will always be challengeable. It is always possible to advance alternative opinions. This is part of the diversity of human thinking. And because there is such variance it is not enough even to search for common opinions shared by all human beings. It is impossible to discover values about which all human beings will agree. Not even seeking to avoid pain and treasuring one's own life can be said always to be universal human values. Athletes seek pain in order to push themselves towards higher performances, and people sometimes commit suicide. However, since these basic values will normally be shared, they do form part of the story about morality.
3. The fundamentals of morality lie in the fact of human existence, in what is naturally human. And it is at this point that the notion of health can be seen to be central to ethics. Human beings have certain physiological and mental potentials common to us all. If these are not allowed to develop in certain people then these people cannot be considered full persons.
   What is a human being for? The only way to answer this question is to give a list of potentials. Some of these, the very potentials on which health work should concentrate, are essential to being a person.
4. Based on the three stages above, and the insight that the achievement of human potential is central to both health and morality in the richest sense (the sense that incorporates the complete iceberg), it is possible to develop an argument that the

fullest degree of morality – or the most ethical intervention – is that which enables persons to achieve the fullest enhancing potentials of which they are capable.

More substance yet needs to be added to this theoretical analysis. In order to be clearer about practical and moral priorities in work for health it is necessary to understand what people – or 'persons' in more technical language – actually are.

# CHAPTER SIX

# What is a Person?

## INTRODUCTION

Like other 'what is?' questions about complex notions, 'what is a person?' is not easy to answer. It ought to be straightforward – 'persons are human beings like you or me' looks the obvious solution – yet it generates several further questions which must be met if a satisfactory account is to be had.

We need a plausible working definition of 'person' to enable us to better understand the nature of those beings for whom health is so important, and to be clear what makes them special. Defining 'person' is a philosophical challenge with significant practical implications. Decisions about whether to switch off life support machines rest on a definition of personhood, for example. They may not depend on this alone, but if a body has no prospect of regaining essential personal characteristics this can be a weighty – and sometimes decisive – consideration.

## THE ARGUMENT OF JOHN HARRIS: TOWARDS A WORKING DEFINITION OF BASIC 'PERSONHOOD'

Like philosophers before him Harris[43] uses 'person' technically, out of line with ordinary use (where it means human beings after infancy). He argues that a person must possess features that make her existence valuable to her. It is not necessary to be human to possess these features (there may be persons on other planets who are not human) nor does it follow that a human being is automatically a person.

Harris quotes John Locke, who also wanted to distinguish persons from other creatures:

> We must consider what 'person' stands for; which, I think is a thinking intelligent being, that has reason and reflection, and can consider itself, the same thinking thing, in different times and places; which it does only by that consciousness which is inseparable from thinking and seems to me essential to it; it being impossible for anyone to perceive that he does perceive.[44]

Locke's point is that although it is impossible for a person to 'perceive that he does perceive' in so far as seeing is concerned – one cannot see oneself seeing – a person can be aware of himself thinking. Locke recognised a condition now generally considered integral to personhood: self-consciousness – the awareness that enables an individual to 'consider itself, the same thinking thing, in different times and places'.

Harris thinks this a necessary condition too, but wishes to expand the concept. For Harris, if a human being is to be classed as a person it not only has to be self-conscious but must have the capacity to value its own life. Hence he unites two conditions: in order for a being to value its own life it has to be aware it has a life to value. This gives a simple definition – a person is 'any being capable of valuing its own existence'.[43]

## 'PERSONS' AND 'FULL HUMAN BEINGS'

Harris discusses an objection offered by Mary Warnock, who resists the use of 'person' on the grounds that it is confusing and could be used as a smokescreen to permit any action on any being so long as it does not count as a person. Warnock prefers the term 'full human being' instead. She thinks membership of the human species the vital moral principle, while Harris favours his version because it avoids 'speciesism' (discrimination between species).

Both 'person' and 'full human being' are meant to offer basic identifying criteria. But neither suggestion goes far enough. Neither stipulates a fulfilled human being – or a 'full person' – yet this is a vital step in the creation of a philosophy of health.

To be a full human being, or to have the capacity to value oneself, is part of what is meant by being a full person, but is not the whole story

Harris and Warnock both recognise the importance of defining what it is to be a valuable living thing. And – Harris' concession to science fiction notwithstanding – both appreciate that a definition is imperative to explain why it is immoral to treat human beings (the vast majority of whom qualify as persons) as objects or with no respect, and to discriminate between beings who are fundamentally equal.

Criteria for personhood are of moral significance because they must be held equally by all. In order to have a firm moral base for medical practice, scientific research, and health care, it is crucial to have a 'bottom line' – a definition of valuable life which effectively prohibits unethical treatment of that life. In the absence of such guidelines a door is left open to those who would ignore the equality of the human condition and exploit people unjustly.

Harris and Warnock clearly share a fundamental concern, yet for the purpose of the present inquiry it is necessary to go further than them. The principle of equal respect for persons is of central importance to health work and rests on the fact that some features of human existence are shared equally by us all. This fact ought to guarantee basic human rights, and is indeed part of the rationale of work for health. However, health work at its richest includes not only the obligation to treat people with equal respect and serve needs first where possible, but also to create and respect autonomy. Therefore it is necessary to construct a notion of 'full personhood' on Harris' basic criteria, in order to recognise these additional responsibilities.

Harris' account of the value of life is made in a book about medical ethics – a tip of the iceberg text to do with hard life and death choices. His basic question is: what is it that makes life valuable at all? His answer refers to an elementary, abstract potential: people have the capacity to value their lives, and do so because they know their lives hold worthwhile future choices. To deny these possibilities to an individual who finds his life valuable is fundamentally wrong. And this is where the argument stops. Indeed this is as far as it is necessary to go for the purpose of helping clinicians and managers make moral decisions according to Harris' conception of morality. But – and this point bears repeating until it gains general acceptance – the ethics of medical work is part of the ethics of health, but is not the whole story. In order to contemplate the ethics of health properly it is necessary to consider what people's future choices might actually be. For Harris' purposes this is not important – all that matters is that there are some rather than no choices for the person. The ethics of health work, on the other hand, is interested in practical detail. The health worker must carefully consider – in theory and in context – the *nature* of the future choices she might enable.

## POTENTIALS

At this point it would perhaps be satisfying to be able to give a list of good and bad human potentials. But things are not this simple. People value different ends, our circumstances are enormously varied, and no two individuals are exactly alike – so a comprehensive list cannot be given. However, when considering persons in the context of health work in its richest sense, an important distinction can be made. It is possible – and necessary for the foundations theory of health – to distinguish between the notion of human potential in the abstract and in practice.

## THE NOTION OF HUMAN POTENTIAL CONSIDERED IN ABSTRACT TERMS

This idea inspires the Harris version of personhood. Even without reference to actual people it is possible to say that all persons and those with the capacity to be persons have potentials. Harris believes the capacity of a being to value its own existence is the most fundamental, but there are others too. For instance, all persons must have the capacity to think and reflect, and all living human beings' bodies must develop: all human beings age so all human beings have biological potential. It can also be said abstractly that some of these potentials will almost always be more desirable than others. For instance, ageing without physical pain is usually preferred to a life of agony. And it is normally thought better that a person values his life because he looks forward to future opportunities, rather than merely because his life exists.

Although it is infuriatingly difficult to specify which potentials should be considered good and which bad, the fact that all persons possess aspects of life in common makes a powerful claim possible. Although the precise degree to which interventions are moral can never be clear, it is nevertheless apparent that to prohibit the achievement of basic potentials in some people and not others is selective dwarfing, and as such is immoral.

## SPECIFIC HUMAN POTENTIALS

Good practical work for health depends upon the empirical investigation of actual potentials (in both individuals and groups). Taking into account the two following conditions – that wherever possible the achievement of a desired potential in an individual should not decrease her future enhancing potentials, and that the achievement of the desired potential should not be at the expense of avoidable dwarfing in other people – it falls to the health worker to consider with the client which of a range of possible potentials should be made reality. Sometimes the decision will be relatively simple. For instance, if a patient has broken his leg the prime consideration will be the restoration of its normal biological potentials. During treatment it may be possible to realise other potentials, dependent on the skill and vision of the health worker concerned. For example, the patient's confidence, knowledge, and understanding might be increased by appropriate kindness, empathy, and education.

In the care of terminally ill people the identification of achievable potentials is often less complicated because time is short and possibilities limited, though their selection can be more painful than in any other area of health work. Much depends on the choice of the patient, and hard decisions sometimes have to be made about the balance between the elimination of pain and the extent to which the patient is able to communicate with those he loves and who love him.

The most baffling choices for health workers face those who deal with people who have a lot of life to come. Such people possess innumerable potentials, only some of which will ever become reality. If health workers are consistently to work in accord with the rich rationale of health work they must take this range into account. Even if the complaint is a simple physical one the best health worker will also seek to explore the client's feelings and future possibilities, viewing his life as a whole. If a competent client does not wish for this sort of intervention then the health worker should stop. However, in principle the health worker has a responsibility to try to discover which potentials might best be actualised. And this requires empirical scrutiny: Does the client need help with a housing problem? Does he need advice about where to find friends? Will he benefit from an opportunity to take a programme of education? Does he have a sporting ambition or talent which is not being expressed? Does he have a creative ability or interest which might be developed by appropriate training and opportunity?

Only if an impoverished view of health work is held are these potentials not thought proper health work. If so, these questions should be asked: why is it important to cure disease – is it so that the morbidity statistics can be improved, or is it so that a person can go on to achieve in his life? How does it make sense to think that the physical aspects of human existence are the most important when the very features that mark off persons from other beings are our capacity for reason, for conceiving intellectually, for valuing our own lives, and for autonomous development?

Work for health is work to create full persons in a much deeper sense than Harris' elementary idea of personhood, and Warnock's notion of a full human being.

# DEWEY'S IDEA OF PERSONAL GROWTH AS THE ONLY TRUE MORAL END

The elegant work of John Dewey adds further substance to the present discussion. John Dewey was one of the few major philosophers to take a deep interest in education, which he considered a central *raison d'être* of philosophy. He believed that 'morals' is 'education', in the general senses of both words. Both notions, he thought, are inseparable from the idea of growth in a child. The end or purpose of the educational process is not something extra to this: 'Growth itself is the only moral end.'[45]

In Dewey's view people are best equipped to realise their individual capacities within a 'democratic society' because:

> All social institutions have a meaning, a purpose. That purpose is to set free and develop *capacities* [my italics] of human individuals without respect to race, sex, class or economic status. And this is all one with saying that the test of their value is the extent to which they educate every individual into the full stature of his possibility. Democracy has many meanings, but if it has a moral meaning, it is found in resolving that the supreme test of all political institutions and industrial arrangements shall be the contribution they make to the all-round growth of every member of society.[45]

Dewey makes an important and comprehensive statement. His words are general and idealistic, but no less valuable for that. His sentiment is entirely in keeping with the spirit of this book. To paraphrase: Dewey's argument is that in a democracy any social institution (whether it is work, school, or the family, for instance) is only moral in so far as it is directed towards the growth, in every possible way, of each unique individual in that society, regardless of race, age, sex, class, or economic status. Any social institution is valuable in proportion to the degree to which it helps every individual, equally, to achieve his or her fullest potential – to flourish – as comprehensively as possible.

Within certain limits[10] this noble aim is precisely what a true health service should aspire to. Interventions aimed at these goals have the most moral intent. Any 'health service' that sets its sights lower than this – for whatever reasons – is not a health service in the most humane sense of the word. Any 'health service' which does not set out to encourage the development of full persons (Dewey's 'flourishing human beings') might exhibit a degree of morality, but not the fullest degree. It will not be the best possible health service, and will be part of a correspondingly less valuable society.

This argument rests on the belief that the single most important principle of a civilised society is that it is designed to provide the same degree of enablement to each of its citizens, regardless of their personal fortune or abilities. This is not a semantic matter. A health service based on these ideals will not only attempt to solve problems of human physique, and will not only make use of the techniques of medicine. Rather it will be a health service which, in Dewey's words will:

> . . . set free and develop the capacities of human individuals without respect to race, sex, class, or economic status . . . [and] educate every individual into the full stature of his possibility . . . Only by being true to the full growth of all individuals who make it up, can society by any chance be true to itself.[45]

## A DIFFICULTY

Once again the problem of discovering a set of values on which all can agree has appeared. It is probable that to those of a socialist or liberal persuasion Dewey's fine rhetoric sounds convincing. Yet it will seem nothing more than words without substance to a person whose views are influenced by the politics of the right.

The question of which potentials should be enabled is clearly a political issue. In a society motivated by individualism it might appear both desirable and appropriate to enable the potential to be self-seeking in another person, if one wishes to see her achieve a higher degree of health than she has at present. But in a society based on a more communitarian rationale it might be neither desirable nor appropriate to enable this particular potential.

## THE POLITICAL ASPECT OF HEALTH CARE

The discussion has returned to the question: what does health mean? The word 'healthy' is so value-laden that a system of health care cannot escape influence from its political environment. A country's health care system can be a mirror, reflecting the degree of morality of the political culture in which it operates.

Different versions of health care can be arranged along a spectrum of types. At the one end health care might be devoted solely to the prevention and elimination of disease and illness, its only function to return bodies to a state where they can again be economically productive, or to make sure that illness does not restrict their abilities to produce. Between the poles health care might treat people as individuals in their own right, but only up to an imprecise and variable limit. And at the other end of the spectrum a health service might be based on the ideology which inspires Dewey, and might limit its resources only when the national budget has been exhausted.

## WHICH OF THESE TYPES IS MOST MORAL IN THE GENERAL SENSE OF MORALITY?

The following answer is given in different form elsewhere in this book. It is restated here for the sake of clarity, and so that the argument can be seen to be progressing coherently.

## ANSWER AND SUMMARY

The answer refers to Grand Thiam, the hypothetical immoral society discussed earlier. It was decided that universal agreement about what is objectively moral cannot be reached because there are so many plausible candidates for the label 'good', and because unique individuals in any of an infinite variety of contexts may not value the same 'goods' to the same degree. However, it was also decided that the deliberate restriction of individual potential to a state less than adulthood is immoral. It is fundamentally wrong to dwarf people physically so that their bodies remain permanently the size of children (what possible justification – in any civilised circumstances – could be offered for such a practice?), so it is at least equally immoral intentionally to disable a person's ability to reason – since it is precisely this facility that distinguishes persons from non-persons. Although it is not possible to go on from this position to state precisely what actions in life are moral, or more moral than others, it *is* possible to assert that the degree of morality achieved will generally be higher the more interventions are opposed to dwarfing.

To conclude, the following points have been made in this chapter. 'Person' is a technical term used by philosophers to describe beings with certain qualities. One of these is a being's ability to value its life, and the possession of this ability implies a basic level of autonomy. These characteristics must be possessed by all persons. And – so long as one accepts that 'person' is a meaningful category – there must be a basic equality amongst all who can be said to be persons. Furthermore, since there is equality of basic characteristics in persons, if we have any moral duties at all we have a duty to treat people equally whenever we can.

In health work it can be enlightening to think of persons more broadly. One of the basic characteristics of personhood is that a person must have some potential for future development. Although the degree and type of future development varies enormously, in every person there exists the possibility to become more of what he could be. The onus rests on health workers to recognise the basic equality of persons, and to strive to ensure their maximum flourishing – paying the fullest attention to the talents and situation of the people concerned. A health system with the goal of enabling human flourishing as equally as possible is surely the most moral system of care.

# Theories of Ethics

Health workers need more than willingness to 'do the right thing' or 'be ethical'. They need ethical tools just as a GP needs her stethoscope to sound a chest, or a surgeon needs physiology and haematology.

Health workers who desire competence in ethical thinking need to understand moral theory. They need to know the strengths and weaknesses of major ethical ideas, and to recognise the types of action each theory is likely to recommend. Like the registrar seeking to gain scalpel skills, health workers need time and experience if they are to work well with their moral instruments.

## INTRODUCTION TO ETHICAL THEORY

### THE ESSENCE OF MORAL REASONING

Moral reasoning – the stamp of civilisation – has been described as a prism[46] able to shine a spectrum of light onto problems. Which light gleams depends on who is doing the thinking. Moral reasoning requires knowledge, intelligence, patience and – from time to time – a will to compromise. Respect for it signifies personal maturity. It is not easy, but done properly moral reasoning is immeasurably better than bullheaded rule-following or mysterious intuition.

### Thinking Ethically

People who appreciate moral reasoning know that rules and principles are both necessary and often conflict. Because of this, edicts must be placed in context to see which are the most appropriate in a given situation. Such a judgement is easiest if the situation is analysed into key elements, the range of alternatives for action made apparent and their pros and cons assessed.

Any course chosen must be justified. This is usually done by appeal to principle or by emphasising the benefit of the expected outcome (or both). Furthermore, the committed moral reasoner does not make ad hoc decisions. She is concerned to choose in the light of previous decisions, and will also want to examine her present solutions with hindsight.

In Chapter Ten the Ethical Grid – an instrument designed to enhance moral reasoning – is introduced as a guide to health workers who would like to be ethically proficient.

It incorporates the elements described above – and more – and is intended as a starting point for personal reflection and public debate. But first it is essential to prepare the ground by reviewing classic theories of Western moral philosophy (some of which the Grid incorporates). The point of this – and of the Grid itself – is not to advocate a particular moral theory (which has been the dominant tradition in recent moral philosophy),[47] but rather to promote a general *way of thinking* amongst health workers.

## A GENERAL DISTINCTION

The major division in Western moral philosophy is between deontology and consequentialism: between the opinion that morality depends on obedience to principles and the view that it rests on the calculation of costs and benefits. As the intricacies of moral philosophy unfold this distinction can seem increasingly blurred. Some deontologists justify their stance on the ground that the consequences of abiding by principles are ultimately desirable, even if they do not maximise utility in the short term. And some consequentialists have claimed we are morally obliged to try to assess the consequences of our actions.

## DEONTOLOGY

(The word deontology is derived from the Greek word deon, and means study of duty.)

The central tenet of deontology is that a moral person must always do her duty. In its purest form deontology holds that a person should perform duties without exception, whatever the consequences. The nature of these duties is open to argument, since there is no principle on which all deontologists agree.

A deontologist might decide to adopt a single overriding duty – for instance, she might advocate that promises should never be broken, or that people should treat others as they wish to be treated themselves. Alternatively the deontologist might adopt a range or hierarchy of duties to guide her actions. If so, in those cases where they conflict, she must decide which duties are most compelling. For example, a deontologist nurse might believe retributive justice (punishment for perceived wrongdoing) should be administered without exception, and that people should always keep promises. If she then promises a youth that whatever he tells her about what is depressing him will be kept confidential, and he tells her he has sold jewellery stolen from his mother, spending the money on fruit machines to feed his addiction to gambling, she has a dilemma. On the one hand she is duty-bound not to break promises, yet on the other she believes wrongdoing should always be penalised. To decide which duties should take precedence in a case such as this the deontologist must come up with a third duty to help her choose between the other two.

Deontological theories contrast with theories which take their guidance from the practical world (two examples are teleological ethics – which maintains that what ought to be done can be decided by studying what is good in fact – and utilitarian ethics, which holds that moral policies can be calculated by assessing happiness levels). Against these, deontological theories argue that the discovery of what is moral is either never, or hardly ever, a matter for empirical research. On the contrary the deontologist – dependent upon how pure a deontologist he is – will argue either that certain obligations and actions are right and good in themselves *regardless* of consequences, or that although it is sensible to consider consequences some duties are nevertheless of supreme and abiding importance.

# TYPES OF DEONTOLOGY

## ACT-DEONTOLOGY

Act-deontology is a rather puzzling version of deontology because it does not define its principles concretely. Indeed act-deontology opposes rule-following, on principle. Sartre and other existentialists have been labelled act-deontologists because they place the focus of moral action not on rules or code books, but on human judgement in the context of each new situation. They assume that however much one situation might appear to resemble another each context and each actor is unique, and so each judgement about each solution should be unique too. A person judging now will be different, in so far as he will have had more experiences, than when he judged then. There are no standards other than the central conviction that everything in morality must rest upon the person who is to decide. Principles are not basic, although they can be considered. Consequences are not basic, although they can be taken into account. The decision-maker is basic. The single obligation of act-deontology is that a person should be true to herself.

### The Advantages of Act-Deontology

Act-deontology is not recommended for health workers enmeshed in the bureaucratic modern world. There must be overt rules and principles of conduct to guide professionals in complex organisations. However, act-deontology's emphasis on being true to oneself whenever moral deliberation is required should not be overlooked, even in the most codified organisations. Indeed, as we shall see, the spirit of act-deontology inspires the Ethical Grid.

Act-deontology draws attention to two important points. Firstly it reminds us that no moral rule can be applied with absolute confidence just because it has turned out well in the past. Each new situation – however similar it might appear to a past one – is unique (as time moves on people and circumstances change inexorably). Surprising things happen and hidden factors can come into play. Therefore it is morally inadequate to stick unthinkingly to rules and convention. Each circumstance is singularly alive and requires the fullest possible attention from the health worker. Simply to do what you have been told, or to carry out your work as if every single aspect of it is routine, is to shut your mind to the importance of yourself and the people in whose lives you intervene.

Secondly, act-deontology explodes the myth that a professional is somehow different from a non-professional. Pompous people think 'professional judgements' are different in kind from those made at home or on holiday. But act-deontology rightly insists that a person should be true to himself in every situation. Being a professional for a time is just another occasion in which authenticity is necessary. There are always choices to be faced: not least the choice between doing what one is contracted to do, and doing what one thinks ought to be done (a common tension for modern health professionals).

## The Disadvantages of Act-Deontology

Act-deontology is inordinately impractical. How can a system of care – or any other system for that matter – be built on a philosophy that advocates arbitrary decisions? While it is true that every situation in life must have distinctive aspects (even if only of time, place, and participants) this is not the same as saying that *everything* about each situation will be unique. Indeed it can be deflating for a person – whether he realises it as a child, an adolescent or in adult life – that there is nothing special about his life other than his own evaluation of it. The human condition is such that we are confronted with problems which are often horribly unique to ourselves, but it is rare for one person to experience a trouble that has not been suffered by many others. Because of this it is necessary to draw up rules – stronger than rules of thumb though not wholly fixed – to deal coherently with human problems.

## RULE-DEONTOLOGY

Rather than insist that a person's moral choosing should depend on how she sees a situation at the time, the rule-deontologist asserts that moral decisions should be based on rules which should be followed whatever the likely outcome. Some rule-deontologists claim their rules are good in themselves while others – in a concession to consequentialism – claim the consequences of not acting according to them will be undesirable.

## The Advantages of Rule-Deontology

The chief advantage of rule-deontology is that the actions of those who espouse it will usually be predictable. Many codes of practice – themselves limited forms of deontology – are in circulation in health services. The principles they contain are usually too general to ensure the predictability deontologists require. However, it would be possible for health service policy-makers to draw up more precise principles, which could be applied according to rule-deontology's intent. For instance, rules such as 'always tell the truth as you know it', 'always keep promises', and 'always respect other people as you would wish to be respected' could be fleshed out by means of detailed examples and case studies, and so become widely recognised principles of practice.

## The Disadvantages of Rule-Deontology

Rule-deontology's main problem is that if a single rule is chosen there will inevitably be occasions when it would be better if it were broken. And if a set of rules is chosen, then although the rules might appear to fit together in the abstract, sooner or later circumstances will reveal clashes between them. The trouble with rule-deontology is that it cannot offer guidance to the health worker who must choose between conflicting rules. Even if the rule-deontologist ranks the rules the first difficulty remains – there will be occasions when it will be much better to override the hierarchy. Indeed there will be occasions on which it is better to ignore even the primary rule, and no further guidance can be offered by the deontological system about when and how to override it.

## SHOULD THE HEALTH SERVICE OPERATE ACCORDING TO GOD-GIVEN RULES?

It is important to think a little about the sorts of argument people of religious faith might advance in favour of the proposition that the health service should be based on supernatural rules.

Many people base their ethics on what they take to be 'God's law'. At their simplest these personal ethics assume an action is right if it has been divinely approved, and wrong if God has forbidden it. The difficulty facing any plan to base a health service on 'God-given' moral principles is that different people understand 'God's law' differently, and of course many others do not accept there is such a thing. Dependent upon which god one recognises (a major hurdle for a health service based in a multi-religious society), or even dependent upon which sections from religious texts are chosen, different moral principles might be followed.

The problems in this respect are similar to those encountered by rule-deontology. They are:

1. Which of the various laws said to be God-given are truly from a deity? Which are most appropriate for a health service, and which deity will confirm this? And if all divine laws are of equal merit, which should a health service adopt?
2. If all divine law is adopted by health workers then, in the inevitable cases of disagreement, how can health workers resolve conflicts?

There are many compassionate health workers who act according to principles derived from religious conviction. And there are equally caring health workers who act on principles derived from other sources. Well-intentioned principles do not require religious justification. Furthermore, religious justification for behaviour is impossible to sustain without all concerned sharing the faith. Since not all health workers and clients have faith it is neither practical nor necessary to base a health service on God-given rules.

## THE INFLUENCE OF IMMANUEL KANT ON ETHICAL THINKING

Kant's ethics forthrightly places duties above consequences. He wanted to construct an objective ethical theory with its source in human reason. Kant thought that certain principles of behaviour could be discovered by any rational human being because they are part of the human make-up. According to Kant, some principles are moral in themselves, and human beings have the capacity to recognise this.

## THE CATEGORICAL IMPERATIVE

The most important feature of Kant's ethics is the 'categorical imperative'. He argued that this imperative is divided into various 'forms', each of which is a duty incumbent upon rational human beings. Kant claimed that any rational human being will be able to see the certainty and necessity of these moral laws by the use of reason.

For present purposes it is not essential to assess all forms of the categorical imperative, or to give a complete account of Kant's argument. However, it is helpful to examine the extent of Kant's emphasis on duties over consequences.

For Kant the only truly moral action is one generated by a pure motive. The truly moral person will do what ought to be done, not after weighing up the pros and cons of what is likely to happen, but simply because she knows she must obey the moral law. Kant wrote:

> To duty every other motive must give place, because duty is a condition of a will good in itself, whose worth transcends everything.[48]

The truly moral act is not influenced by self-interest, nor by consideration of social benefit. The moral person does her duty because she sees she must.

## THE ESSENCE OF KANT'S CATEGORICAL IMPERATIVE

The central principle of the categorical imperative is familiar to several movements, both religious and atheistic, and rests on the belief that human beings are entitled to equal consideration. Although we obviously have different abilities and constantly find ourselves in changing circumstances, we have shared characteristics sufficient to warrant the conclusion that 'we are all in the same boat'. Given this it follows that no moral person will act towards any other in a way he himself would not wish to be treated, a conclusion encapsulated in Kant's first formulation of the categorical imperative:

> Act only on that maxim which you can at the same time will to be universal law.

In other words, act like this only if you wish anyone else in like circumstances to do the same. Before you deliberately say something hurtful, before you steal, before you decide no one will know you haven't paid your coffee money at work, or before you do nothing when you could have done good, you must genuinely will that your action become universal law.

More specifically, Kant's ethical theory can be divided into three parts. The first is the general dictum discussed briefly above. The second adds more substance to the imperative, and the third part unites the other two.

The three parts are:

1. *If you wish to act morally act as if your action in each circumstance is to become law for everyone, yourself included, in the future.*
2. *If you wish to act morally always treat other human beings as 'ends in themselves' and never merely as 'means'.*

By this Kant meant that it is unethical to treat people as if they are objects – mere tools to be used to further your own ambitions and ends. It is morally essential to recognise that all other people have ends of their own. They have emotions, hopes, and anxieties just as you do, and just as you wish to be respected, other people's feelings and aspirations should be respected equally. According to Kant it is fundamentally immoral to exploit a person without considering her an end in her own right.

3. *If you wish to act morally always act as a member of a community where all the other members of that community are 'ends', just as you are.*

## WHY DID KANT CHOOSE THESE PRINCIPLES?

*If you wish to act morally act as if your action in each circumstance is to become law for everyone, yourself included, in the future.*

Kant considered it a natural instinct (i.e. a reaction not based upon reason) for people to be self-interested (unless they are enlightened by the 'moral law'). Conversely, the first principle holds that an essential feature of morality is impartiality in the subject. If a person always operates according to the first principle it becomes fundamentally wrong for that person to make an exception of himself. In other words, when considering how to act it is wrong to believe yourself to be of any more merit than anyone else.

The first principle does not state specifically which sorts of action are good or bad. Instead it forces the actor to examine her moral conscience every time she contemplates an action. If she decides she would not like what she is intending to do to someone else to happen to her, or if she will enjoy what she is doing for herself but would not welcome the consequences if everyone behaved in that way, then according to this principle she must conclude that the proposed action is morally wrong.

*If you wish to act morally always treat other human beings as 'ends in themselves' and never merely as 'means'.*

This principle is intended to add more substance to the first. Kant was not so idealistic as to hope that in each everyday dealing we will consider the wishes and goals of others. It would be bizarre to inquire into the life history of shop assistants met only once, for example. In this case, or in the case of an employer and employee where the relationship depends upon a financial contract, it is inevitable that people will treat each other as means. Kant saw nothing wrong with this provided people are not treated always as means. To be moral in an interaction you must respect the other person's ends when appropriate. For example, if the shop assistant breaks down in tears and begs for your help then you should not treat her as a means.

To treat a person 'as an end' is to recognise that the person has his own purposes, just as you have yours. The secret is to imagine your own death. Imagine how much will be lost when you die – a lifetime of hopes, fears, imaginings, achievements, and introspection will disappear. A world will expire. Think of other people with this in mind and you can hardly fail to understand what is meant by the advice to treat them as ends. Slavery, for example, is a clear moral wrong according to this way of thinking.

When a person is enslaved he is, to quote Aristotle, treated as nothing more than a living tool.

*If you wish to act morally always act as a member of a community where all the other members of that community are 'ends', just as you are.*

The idea behind Kant's third principle is that a moral agent should act as a member of a community of persons, all of whom are just as able to make moral decisions as the agent herself. The implication of this, and the link with the other two principles, is that each member of the community should respect the desires of others and allow them freedom of decision. Each will recognise that everyone can and should behave as if they, as a result of their choices and actions, are legislating for everyone else.

## Politics and Ethics

Certain political conclusions follow from Kant's ethical theories. The association between ethics and politics is not always noticed, even though political implications are bound to ensue from any prescriptive ethical theory. The Ethical Grid is part of such a theory, and so has political consequences for health work and the health service. This theory, like Kant's, is a democratic ethic which defines 'a democratic society' as one in which every one of its members can have a say in how it develops. Kantian ethics requires liberty, since each citizen should be as free as possible to choose for herself. It also requires fraternity in the sense that each person should consider himself a member of a moral community – a member of a community shared by others with equal moral rights and responsibilities.

# SOME PROBLEMS WITH KANT'S THEORY OF ETHICS

There is a significant difficulty with Kant's central doctrine:

> Act only on that maxim which you can at the same time will to be universal law.

Kant seems to have intended it to cause people to stop to think before acting. A person who wishes to be moral in Kant's sense might, for example, pause before breaking a promise – perhaps a promise to his wife – to consider whether he would wish that the maxim (that it is right for husbands to break promises to their wives) on which he was about to act should become a universal law. Kant was convinced the moral actor would conclude that he could not will this. What would the institution of marriage be like in this case? For Kant, the austere moral philosopher, there could be no exceptions. He could not conceive how any rational person could universalise a maxim that it is right to break promises. Consequently, it followed for Kant that it must always be wrong to break a promise to one's wife.

What are modern health workers to make of Kant's moral philosophy? It might seem that Kant's work can help provide a structured code of practice, allowing each health worker some responsibility for decision-making (since each could imagine herself legislating universally). But this expectation is dashed when one realises the severity of Kant's advice.

His imperatives are unyielding. But in the complex health world the ability to be flexible, to be able to make rapid judgements about complicated ethical problems under pressure and sometimes to arrive at sensible compromises, is essential to the best health work. A little thought shows it can often be better to make an exception to a moral rule. There are, for instance, occasions when a strong argument can be made that to break a promise to one's wife or husband is the best moral choice. Perhaps you solemnly vowed that if she ever again came home after midnight without letting you know, you would throw her suitcases, clothes, cat, and back catalogue of *Harper's and Queen* out the window. And it turns out her car and cell 'phone *truly* have broken down in the wilds.

But Kant's position is relentlessly uncompromising. There can be no exceptions to the duty to keep a promise, or to tell the truth, or whatever else the duty is. If it is right to keep a promise in one instance then it must be right to keep a promise in any other. Moreover, Kant took little account of the consequences of actions. Although he must have believed that doing one's duty causes desirable consequences, this thought seems to have occurred only on an intellectual plane.

It is not difficult to think of exceptions to the sorts of duty Kant imagined should be moral law. Consider the duty to act on the maxim 'tell the truth', which Kant thought the rational person must will. Imagine that a badly injured man regains consciousness in a hospital bed. He is critically ill and fighting for his life after a road accident. It is hard to see how it makes moral sense to tell him the truth – that his wife and three daughters have been killed – until his condition is no longer critical, and the news unlikely to endanger his life (though it would be a different matter if he were about to die).

Consider too the maxim 'minimise harm', where a psychiatrist is considering whether or not to treat compulsorily a woman who has been making intimidating threats. In this case the problem is that it is unclear what the moral legislator would be universalising. In circumstances like this what counts as harm and which harms are worse than others are matters open to question – so Kant's dictum is not only inflexible but impossible to apply specifically where matters are open to interpretation. The best a legislator might will is that people should act to minimise harm *as they see it*.

## FURTHER OBJECTIONS

The earlier part of this book has shown that the nature of ethics is indistinct and disputable, and that there are alternative senses in which morality can be used. Because Kant did not make the difference between morality and immorality exact, it is possible to interpret his general commandments in different ways. In the absence of a practical definition it is possible to offer justifications for behaviour which many theories of ethics would not accept. For instance, a person might will that the maxim 'no one should steal' should become a universal law, and do so entirely out of self-interest. The person who wills this might have a large house and money in the bank, and be interested only in maintaining this position. Only 'egotism' offers a similar account of morality. Clearly Kant did not intend it, but by leaving the details up to moral agents to decide it seems he must accept this result.

Kant wanted to argue that people should not make deceitful promises, and then break them to suit their own ends. However, even the duty not to make deceitful promises (or not to break promises) is not obviously the most moral course of action in every circumstance. For example, perhaps money has been lent by a corrupt government which tortures dissidents, and the debtor decides to use it to fund a campaign against torture.

It would be heartening to be able to agree with Kant that whatever the consequences it is morally important to abide by a pure motive to do one's duty, but such a stance is impossible to prove in this world. Being moral is surely a more complex and burdensome responsibility than sticking to abstract duties. Striving to be moral is difficult – it requires good intentions but also demands thought, foresight, logic, detachment, and integrity – human qualities just as precious as the supposed faculty of pure reason.

The principle of ends offers incomplete advice about how to act morally. If a person attempts to adopt the principle of ends in real life he will inevitably be faced with situations where he will affect people whom he will not be able to treat as ends. If, for instance, a scarce resource can be offered only to a proportion of those who could benefit from it, then the actor who is in a position to distribute it, and who wishes to treat all potential recipients as ends, faces an impossible task. She might, for instance, be an admissions tutor at university, and dearly wish to admit all who have applied to her degree course. But places are limited and only some applicants can have their wishes respected, and so be treated as ends. The remainder, no matter how kind the letter of rejection, must be discarded as if they are of no account, just because life is often like that.

If a person fails to treat as ends all those he might have treated as ends, then he has offended against the moral law as Kant perceived it. What is more, the principle of ends offers no criterion by which to decide who should be treated as ends, when not everyone can.

## WHAT FEATURES SHOULD HEALTH WORKERS NOTE MOST OF ALL ABOUT KANT'S ETHICAL THEORY?

The core of Kant's moral philosophy is that once a person is in tune with his moral conscience it is a relatively simple matter to act in the most moral way. For Kant moral issues are not complex or insoluble – ethics is not cerebral perpetual motion – rather it is possible for a person to be consistently moral, and moral in exactly the same way as all other persons within the moral community, by using the faculty of reason. Through reflection and introspection it is possible, according to Kant, to discover laws. It is not enough simply to obey rules because it is legal or because it is part of your job (those who carry out immoral instructions from their superiors can have no moral defence for their actions in Kant's view). Personal motive is crucial. It is up to individuals to discover the pure motives (the moral path) for themselves, often in spite of external pressure to the contrary. Health workers who insist on following instructions and codes because it is expedient for them to do so may well find something in Kant's work to move them to revise their opinions.

Universalisability is another lynchpin of Kant's moral philosophy. It is important for health workers to note that this idea rests on the notion that all people are equal in crucial respects, whatever their position and circumstances in life. Consequently, at least according to Kant, it is fundamentally immoral to act towards one person or group of persons in situation X whilst acting differently towards other persons also in situation X, whatever the external justification. What is so impressive about Kant's work is his insistence that all people should be treated as ends acting within a community in which all other people have equal status as moral agents, or potential moral agents, and are entitled to equal respect because of this – whatever their economic status or whatever their age or physical condition. (Actually there were some exceptions. Kant thought criminals should be punished because, through their crimes, they sacrifice the right to be treated as ends – and this part of his argument is inconsistent with the rationale of work for health presented in this book.)

In sum, Kant prizes individual responsibility and believes that people ought to be treated as equals, since we all share the uniquely human ability to reason morally. This fact transcends our material differences. What is perhaps less useful to health workers is his idea that individual responsibility and freedom to make the best moral judgements stops when universalisable rules are discovered. In the fraught world of health care there are cases in which the human interest is best served by suspending 'moral laws'.

Finally, the most significant inadequacy of Kant's theory – an inadequacy health workers ignore at their peril – is its underemphasis on consequences. In the real world it is no defence, either morally or legally, to say that what was done was done out of a pure motive to be moral. Considerations of logic, probability of outcome, and actual outcome must enter the picture when the degree of morality is assessed.

A more complete view of morality comes into play when the consequences are considered. The ethical realm incorporates much more than pure motive – just like in law where conspiracy to murder (intent to murder) and actual murder (where the consequence is that life is lost) are different crimes with different punishments. And beyond the legal sphere, wanting to be kind to another person is not the same as actually being kind to her. Actually being kind to a person surely shows a higher degree of morality than meaning to, but never getting around to it.

# THE ETHIC OF CONSEQUENCES

## WHAT IS CONSEQUENTIALISM AND WHAT IS UTILITARIANISM?

For the sake of clarity it is important to explain the difference between consequentialism and utilitarianism. Consequentialism is the more global ethical theory, utilitarianism its major subset. However, such are the similarities between the two that it is sufficient to introduce consequentialism, and to direct the majority of the discussion to utilitarianism – the best known term.

## CONSEQUENTIALISM

On the face of it consequentialism is a straightforward doctrine, apparently diametrically opposed to Kant's version of deontology. In its most radical form consequentialism holds that the rightness or wrongness of an act should be judged solely on whether its consequences produce more benefits than disadvantages, the nature of 'benefit' and 'disadvantage' having been defined beforehand by the consequentialist. A consequentialist decides how to act by assessing the likely outcomes of her proposed action, and judges the morality of what she has or has not done according to how her action turns out.

## UTILITARIANISM

Utilitarianism is classically associated with the goal of happiness or pleasure. However, moral philosophers have come to think such a simple measure rather crude, and other measures of utility are now considered legitimate. Indeed it is now rather artificial to distinguish between utilitarianism and consequentialism.

Unlike deontological theory, utilitarianism does not depend upon principles and commandments – it does not assume that there are naturally right things to do. Utilitarianism is not concerned with motives for actions, but with the results of actions. At its simplest the utilitarian prescription is this: a person ought always to act so as to produce the greatest balance of good over bad.

But what is good and what is bad? The earliest form of utilitarianism defined 'the good' as 'pleasure' or 'happiness'. The 'greatest happiness principle' of Jeremy Bentham (who, along with Mill, is most usually associated with utilitarianism) states that a person should attempt to achieve 'the greatest good, or greatest happiness, of the greatest number' (though this formula does not make it clear whether the good should be distributed as widely and equally as possible, or is best concentrated in the hands of a few). One alternative definition of the utilitarian good was proposed by G. E. Moore who thought, presumably on the basis of his own preferences, that the central human goods were personal relationships and aesthetic experiences.[49]

But whatever the definition of good and evil these goods and evils must be *measurable*. It is crucial to utilitarianism (the forebear of economics) that a cost-benefit calculation can be made. A judgement about what to do cannot depend on opinion only, rather it must be possible to work out an answer according to standards laid down beforehand.

Importantly, utilitarianism does not hold that the highest good is the good of the self (which would be a form of egotism) but insists that the person working out what to do (the moral agent) must be considered of equal importance to everyone else in the assessment. As Mill argues:

> The utilitarian standard of what is right in conduct is not the agent's own happiness but that of all considered. As between his own happiness and that of others, utilitarianism requires him to be as strictly impartial as a disinterested and benevolent spectator.[50]

In other words utilitarianism requires that a person should *sacrifice* his self-interest if this is likely to bring about an increase in the general good.

# TYPES OF UTILITARIANISM

## ACT-UTILITARIANISM

Act-utilitarianism states that in any situation a person should, if he is to do the right thing, assess which of the actions open to him is most likely to produce the greatest balance of good over evil (however defined). It falls to the act-utilitarian, in each case he faces, to ask: 'What effect will my action have on the amount of good in the world?' Where a deontologist might think he has a moral duty to keep promises in all circumstances, an act-utilitarian will not take this for granted. Instead, in the light of the unique and specific prevailing conditions, he will weigh up the pros and cons of keeping the promise, always giving the fullest possible attention to a consideration of the likely outcome. If keeping the promise does not seem likely to produce a balance of good over evil then – according to act-utilitarianism – he is justified in breaking it.

Act-utilitarian problem-solving need not be quite as ad hoc as this since act-utilitarians must also access the likely effects (short and long term) on other people, caused by a glib breaking of a promise for the sake of expedience. And it may be that the decrease in general levels of integrity is not considered a price worth paying.

Act-utilitarianism can best be described as a form of opportunism. It does not endorse rules other than the requirement to calculate (although there is a modified form of act-utilitarianism which permits 'rules of thumb' based on past experiences – to avoid having to deliberate afresh every time). If, on balance, the outcome of your intended action is likely to be good, then do it! Do it whatever it is, even if it is stealing, or lying, or causing physical harm, or destroying someone emotionally, or blackmailing, or breaking the law of the land, or murdering someone, or betraying a friend. If you think your action will produce more good than evil in the end, then that is what you should do.

## WHAT FEATURES OF ACT-UTILITARIANISM ARE RELEVANT FOR HEALTH WORKERS?

First, it is difficult to imagine any health system suggesting that its staff become act-utilitarians. For example, enthusiastic converts might seek to justify a lower standard of care – or even non-voluntary euthanasia – for old people occupying beds that could be used to care for younger people. Such discrimination, although possibly justifiable in utilitarian terms, is not work for health.

There is a further practical problem. The act-utilitarian must assess, in each and every case, the likely ratio of good and evil. Yet this requirement is unrealistic in the urgent health care world. What is needed is a way of reflection that does not demand calculation afresh in every case, yet which nevertheless offers individuals the opportunity to think for themselves.

This focus on individual responsibility is the main advantage of act-utilitarianism. Just as act-deontology claims that a person has a basic duty to reflect on the array of principles available, so act-utilitarianism offers a compelling reminder that inherited rules of practice need not be obeyed in all cases. Given rules might be disobeyed if the health worker calculates it is better to do so. Sometimes sticking to the rules might produce unacceptable consequences (perhaps the house rule is to offer only cursory explanations of treatment).

## GENERAL UTILITARIANISM

This version of utilitarianism advocates neither unique responses nor rules. Instead, general utilitarianism requires a potential actor to ask, 'What if everyone were to do what I propose to do?' For example, a doctor of medicine about to deceive a patient about his condition should ask himself what the consequences would be if everyone hid information they think other people do not want to hear.

General utilitarianism is uncomplicated. Most people have said disapprovingly, 'What if everybody did that?' and there is worth in this common dictum. However, as far as health care is concerned the theory is a little incomplete, and is best used as a stimulus to thought. For instance, recall the case of Diane the Health Visitor (Chapter Four), whose aim was not to produce the highest possible proportion of child immunisations, but to enable parents to weigh up the pros and cons of vaccinating their children. For Diane the highest priority was not a possible decrease in disease and illness, but a possible increase in the level of education. The response to Diane, 'but what if everyone did that?' is commonplace amongst community nurses who argue, for instance, that if all health visitors saw themselves as remedial educators rather than medical workers this might have bad consequences for the health service, whose level of future funding depends in part upon the sort of 'performance indicator' good immunisation rates produce. And how would general practitioners react to an army of rebel 'nurse educators'?

However, 'what if everybody did that?' is not always a damning response. It is equally possible for nurses who think like Diane to ask 'what if everybody did that?' of those who think of immunisation work as a sales campaign.

## RULE-UTILITARIANISM

Echoing rule-deontology, rule-utilitarianism argues that obedience to rules, not personal judgement, is fundamental to morality. But where rule-deontology applies preordained rules, rule-utilitarianism holds that rules of conduct are to be worked out by discovering which, if always adhered to, will produce the greatest balance of good over evil. The justification for rules is in their utility rather than their purity, but this proviso apart, there are marked similarities between rule-deontology and rule-utilitarianism.

In contrast to act-utilitarianism, where it can be acceptable to maintain rules – but only as a general guideline – a rule-utilitarian wants to keep a rule which will produce the greatest good in the long run. So, for example, a rule-utilitarian might calculate that the best consequences result from obedience to the rule 'always tell the truth'.

The difference between act-utilitarianism and rule-utilitarianism can be demonstrated like this:

You are a health education officer. You are aware that your friend has been stealing from the stationery store regularly for the last two years. Most people you know have done something like this in the past, and it is not usually regarded as a serious crime. It is seen more as a perk of the job. However, one day your manager asks you a direct question:

'Has Albert stolen the coloured duplicating paper meant for those posters to publicise our "learning communities for a holistic millennium" meeting?'

You know he has and you know also that if you tell the truth your friend's job will be in serious danger.

It is likely, although of course not certain, that an act-utilitarian would say utility demands that a lie be told to help Albert and his family – after all it is only a minor misdemeanour and will perhaps be the jolt he needs to stop – while a rule-utilitarian would tell the truth on the ground that it is better in the long run, even though there might be temporary benefit in telling a lie.

## WHAT FEATURES OF RULE-UTILITARIANISM ARE RELEVANT FOR HEALTH WORKERS?

Rule-utilitarian health workers use rules derived from careful consideration of past costs and benefits. Their principal problem is a difficulty for all varieties of utilitarianism (including health economics). That is, there may be occasions on which their policy creates an excess of good over evil for a population as a whole, but does not distribute it fairly. Thus a principle of justice (that all social goods ought to be distributed equally) is undermined by utilitarianism. The British Labour Party argued that just such a calculation was made by the Tory Government of the 1980s. There is considerable utility in maintaining a high level of unemployment (unions are kept under control because there is endemic fear of unemployment, output increases, house costs decrease and there is an increase in the standard of living for those in permanent, well-paid jobs). The majority enjoy benefit (and so are more likely to vote for you next time) while the minority suffer, and on utilitarian terms this is fair enough.

To take a health service example, it might promote utility to move non-dangerous mentally ill people from hospitals to the community. It might save money and it might help some patients become happier and better adjusted, but if such a policy is carried out without room for exceptions then there will inevitably be some patients, relatives, and carers who suffer (many mental health workers and consumers say that exactly this has been the effect of over-zealous de-institutionalisation in recent years).

Here is a classic illustration of utilitarianism's clash with justice as fairness:

> . . . let us imagine that the happiness of the whole human race were to be immeasurably increased – poverty eliminated, brotherhood achieved, disease conquered . . . but the condition is that one man, his life mysteriously prolonged, is to be kept involuntarily in a state of continuous and agonising torture. According to the utilitarian criterion, which measures the rightness of an act by its results, it would seem that the argument is justified . . . the net balance of the utilitarian moral scale would have to point in the direction of maximum happiness and away from the eternal agony of the single suffering man. But most people who consider the proposed bargain feel that there is something terribly wrong with it.[51]

A further general problem with utilitarianism arises because utilitarians must claim that any action is right so long as it brings about favourable consequences – even if the intention of the actor is clearly evil. For example, imagine that through deliberate and excessive cost-cutting a private cosmetic surgeon has disfigured 50 patients, two of whom were driven to suicide as a result. The malpractice comes to light and the doctor is struck off the medical register, compensation paid to all victims and – most important of all – a thorough policing of cosmetic surgery advertisers is carried out in future. This ensures such malpractice cannot reoccur, thus sparing potentially thousands of people unnecessary trauma. Since this is the outcome the utilitarian must define the corrupt doctor's actions as moral, despite his immoral intent.

To give an example beyond the medical field, in 1996 Martyn Bryant went on a crazy rampage in Port Arthur in Tasmania, killing 35 people and seriously damaging the lives of thousands of their friends and relatives. Bryant's intent cannot possibly be described as moral yet, because Australia's gun laws (and those of some other countries) have been stiffened up and police monitoring of dangerous people made more rigorous, his actions will probably increase happiness in the long term. Such incongruities as these are hard to reconcile unless utilitarians are prepared to dilute their ideas with aspects of other moral theories. But if they do this then their approaches can no longer be described as utilitarian.

(Note: it would be wrong to think of deontologists and consequentialists as tribespeople, always acting in accord with the dictates of their preferred moral theory. In reality those who espouse technical ethics treat the subject like a game. For the sake of argument or prestige a philosopher will sometimes defend a position to the hilt – for instance, she might argue that in every possible circumstance her idiosyncratic version of rule-utilitarianism is always the most moral option – but rarely, if ever, will she carry this position into everyday life.)

# THE FOUR PRINCIPLES APPROACH

Two decades ago two American academics, Tom Beauchamp and Jim Childress, published the 'four principles approach' to medical ethics.[52,53,54] This idea has proved widely influential in both teaching and writing about medical ethics, particularly amongst clinicians and nurses with little or no philosophical knowledge. I have lost count of the papers I have read which state – almost always without argument or elucidation – that '. . . the four principles of medical/health care/bioethics are beneficence, non-maleficence, respect for autonomy and justice'.

Beauchamp describes the principles more fully as:

1. Beneficence (the obligation to provide benefits and balance benefits against risks).
2. Non-maleficence (the obligation to avoid the causation of harm).
3. Respect for autonomy (the obligation to respect the decision-making capacities of autonomous persons).
4. Justice (obligations of fairness in the distribution of benefits and risks).[53]

The four principles idea is deceptively simple. By using these principles, either singly or in combination, a doctor is supposed to be able to give a satisfactory answer to any moral problem he comes across in his work. He may need 'additional interpretation and specification'[53] and further rules such as ' "Don't Kill" and "Tell the Truth" ',[53] but the four principles are thought by their advocates to provide an adequate framework for all moral deliberation in health care.

Raanan Gillon, long-time editor of the *Journal of Medical Ethics* and a four principles devotee, offers fulsome support to Beauchamp and Childress:

> In brief, the four principles plus scope approach claims that whatever your personal philosophy, politics, religion, moral theory or life stance, you will find no difficulty in committing yourself to four *prima facie* moral principles plus a concern for their scope of application . . . these . . . can be seen to encompass most if not all of the moral issues that arise in health care (I am increasingly inclined to believe that the approach can, if sympathetically interpreted, be seen to encompass *all* moral issues, not merely those arising in health care) . . . '*Prima facie*' . . . means that the principle is binding unless it conflicts with another moral principle – if it does then you have to choose between them. The four principles approach does not claim to provide a method for doing so . . . [W]hat the principles . . . approach *can* provide is a common set of moral commitments, a common moral language, and a common set of moral issues to be considered in particular cases, before coming to your own answer, using your preferred moral theory or other approach to choosing between these principles when they conflict . . .[54]

Beauchamp affirms Gillon's understanding of *prima facie*:

> [the four principles] . . . are *prima facie*: they are always binding *unless* they conflict with obligations expressed in another moral principle, in which case a balancing of the demands of the two principles is necessary. In this event, further specification is required of the precise commitments of the guidelines for the special circumstance(s). Which principle overrides in a case of conflict will depend on the particular context, which is likely to have unique features.[53]

Beauchamp admits that:

> . . . some have severely criticised the four-principles approach as a 'mantra of principles', meaning that the principles have functioned for some adherents like a ritual incantation of norms repeated with little reflection or analysis.[53]

and cites three criticisms in particular:

> Gert and Clouser bring the following accusations . . . (1) the 'principles' are little more than checklists or headings for lists of values worth remembering, and so the principles have no deep moral substance and do not produce directive guidelines for moral conduct; (2) principle analyses fail to provide a theory of justification or a theory that ties the principles together so as to generate clear, coherent, specific rules, with the consequence that the principles and so-called derivative rules are *ad hoc* constructions without systematic order; (3) these *prima facie* principles must often compete in difficult circumstances, yet the underlying account is unable to decide how to adjudicate the conflict in particular cases and unable theoretically to deal with a conflict of principles.[53]

Astonishingly Beauchamp not only does not deny that these are problems, but is quite unable to offer any answer to them. His only defence is that they are also problems for anyone else who uses principles or rules. He then uses a dismally ubiquitous academic's ploy – he is unable to fortify his own position so he attacks his critics' thinking instead.

The four principles approach is manifestly empty, and has achieved its great popularity as a direct result. Because the principles lack detail – and since their adherents' attempted justifications swiftly collapse into waffle – they can be used by almost anyone to defend almost anything, and have a special appeal to those for whom existing arrangements are good. For such lucky men and women the principles will very likely seem to:

> . . . encompass most if not all of the moral issues that arise in health care (and may) be seen to encompass *all* moral issues . . .[54]

because they will rarely if ever have reason to question them.

The exquisite extract below surely establishes waffle as an art-form:

> In this event, further specification is required of the precise commitments of the guidelines for the special circumstance(s). Which principle overrides in a case of conflict will depend on the particular context, which is likely to have unique features.[53]

Moreover – despite the waffly camouflage – Gillon and Beauchamp's use of *'prima facie'* is inescapably authoritarian. Here is Gillon's version again:

> . . . whatever your personal philosophy, politics, religion, moral theory or life stance, you will find no difficulty in committing yourself to four *prima facie* moral principles plus a concern for their scope of application . . . these . . . can be seen to encompass most if not all of the moral issues that arise in health care . . . *'Prima facie'* . . . means that the principle is binding unless it conflicts with another moral principle – if it does then you have to choose between them. The four principles approach does not claim to provide a method for doing so.[54]

Let's look at this a little more closely. We are asked to accept – no, we are told – that each of the four principles is objectively binding on us – only if there are conflicts can a principle be disregarded, and then only if it is overridden by one of the other three. The ethical question is thus never – do I accept the social arrangements which generated this ethical problem (not enough money for care of the elderly, for instance)? – and always – which moral truth should I bring to bear to offer the best solution in the circumstances I accept as given?

Gillon's claim is so astounding it is hard to believe it has been taken seriously:

> . . . whatever your personal philosophy, politics, religion, moral theory or life stance, you will find no difficulty in committing yourself to four *prima facie* moral principles plus a concern for their scope of application . . .[54]

As a matter of fact this is nonsense. If you are a Marxist, or a Sartrian, or a utilitarian, or a different sort of deontologist, or a cultural relativist (to name but a few) you will have an insurmountable difficulty accepting the four principles because they will not be part of the moral theory you espouse.

Gert and Clouser's criticisms are, of course, spot on. In addition, each of the principles is open to interpretation so wide that it is unintelligible to state 'I am following principle X' without further explanation of what you take X to mean. And if you do bother to spell out what you mean more exactly you will find you have gone beyond the principles anyway – intelligent reflection on moral priorities renders the four principles redundant.

But the worst problem with the four principles approach is that it does not explain *why* one should follow it. Of course it is a helpful teaching tool and can be a useful starting point for analysis, but its proponents never say why respect for autonomy, for instance, should be binding (either in health care or in life in general). It is not self-evident that it should. Indeed in many areas of our lives our autonomy is not respected – and not just in those areas (like road traffic law) where we might harm others (I'd like better wages, my MP to represent my views not his, and all doctors to act on my philosophy, but it doesn't happen). In order to explain why one should choose the four principles matters of meaning and purpose have to be addressed – philosophical questions must be determinedly pursued in order to develop an underlying theory capable of supporting moral conclusions.

Beauchamp, Childress and Gillon have got it lamentably wrong. Nebulous principles generally acceptable to well-heeled Western liberals do no more than offer conclusions (a) open to wide interpretation and (b) acceptable only to those who agree with them in the first place ('justice' is a prime example, and is discussed in the following section). In order to engage in serious moral reflection it is necessary first to have a sustained and specific understanding of the importance of your enterprise. This way there can be constructive disagreement with those who hold alternative theories, key words such as 'autonomy' and 'justice' will have clear and distinctive meaning, and there will be no need for the hopeless assumption that everyone is bound by obviously contestable ideas. Given strong theories of purpose controversy can take place where it ought to – over the meaning and importance of practical health and social goals.

# JUSTICE

## WHAT IS JUSTICE?

This question is as difficult as 'what is health?' The only certainty is that a definitive answer is impossible. As with 'health' there are several meaningful uses of the word, all of which are sometimes claimed as the true interpretation. However, none of them should be allowed to dominate because it is only in multiplicity that the richest sense of justice can be gleaned.

Justice is commonly thought of in two ways: justice as fairness and justice as appropriate punishment for wrongdoing. Justice as fairness is violated when people equal in all relevant aspects are nevertheless treated unequally. Justice as appropriate punishment for wrongdoing is known as retributive justice, but is not of concern in the present inquiry.

## THREE VERSIONS OF JUSTICE AS FAIRNESS

Justice as fairness can be subdivided in three interesting ways – all of which are undoubtedly part of the notion of justice overall, but only one of which is fundamental to a true health service. The three types are: to each according to his rights, to each according to what he deserves, and to each according to his need. Of these, only the final dictum informs the richest sense of work for health (see Miller[55] for a full analysis of this topic).

The expression 'to each according to his rights' is essentially contractual justice. For example, if a person agrees to labour for a specified sum of money it is his right – and it is just – that his employer pays him his due (so long as the worker has abided by the conditions of the contract). The phrase 'to each according to what he deserves' is used to justify meritocracies, in which those who work the hardest or most successfully gain the best rewards. If a woman puts in long hours building up a business then, if there is to be justice in this sense, she should reap the harvest of her endeavours. Similarly, if a man strives diligently to obtain good university degrees, accruing debt and sacrificing the opportunity to earn more outside university then – according to this under-standing of justice – it is only fair that he should eventually be accorded the status and earning power his studying and application merit.

Both these concepts are highly contentious. For example, in Western countries people have equal rights to own property, but some people are hugely rich while others have nothing. These inequalities are so marked that it is often argued that an alternative principle of justice (usually to each according to need) should override 'to each according to his right', at least in exceptional cases. Likewise with justice as desert, which is called into question by considerations such as this: perhaps the young man who has worked hard at university does in a sense deserve to enjoy the benefits of his dedication. But this is tempered by the knowledge that he has been privileged to have been able to attend a good university in the first place. Not everyone can secure a university place – and far fewer are able to find a place at a decent institution. Because they enjoy a sound upbringing – which brings early access to books, a wide parental vocabulary, and positive peer pressures – middle-class children have a better chance of attending a good university than their working-class contemporaries, even though their talents might be equivalent.

Of course the above discussion is superficial, and it may also be argued that justice as 'to each according to his need' has inadequacies at least as serious. However, it should be a founding principle of a true health service. Indeed it is already embraced by health workers who wish to help anyone overcome physical and mental problems – whoever they are and whatever they have done.

True work for health is not driven primarily by the wish to ensure that contracts are honoured (although this is sometimes important), nor does it offer care only to those considered to have earned it, rather it concentrates first and foremost on people's needs (within certain limits)[1] whether these are food or warmth or shelter or surgery or kindness or advice or education or love. True health care is informed by a notion of justice which regards the fulfilment of need, equally and without unwarranted discrimination, as a fundamental premise.

## A DEVELOPED NOTION OF JUSTICE – RAWLS AND JUSTICE AS FAIRNESS

Although justice cannot be comprehensively analysed in this book it is such an important notion that it is worth introducing John Rawls' work, meant to provide an elaborate method through which to ensure just social organisation.[56]

## THE JUST SOCIETY ARISING FROM A VEIL OF IGNORANCE

Rawls' theory is complicated. However, at bottom it insists that the unequal distribution of desirable qualities like power, wealth, and income is unjust, unless the inequality works to benefit the worst-off citizens.

In order to demonstrate the strength of this claim Rawls asks us to imagine ourselves in a hypothetical situation, in which we are a free, logical, yet disinterested being about to enter into a social contract with everyone else. The most intriguing feature of Rawls' proposal is that none of the parties to the contract knows what or where she will be in the system once it has taken shape. The contract is to be made behind a veil of ignorance which completely conceals the actual place and condition of all involved. The contractor might be male or female, young or old, employer or employee, rich or poor, diseased or not.

After asking us to imagine this pre-contractual situation Rawls asks: which principles should govern social arrangements behind the veil? Or in other words: which principles inform the just society? It is well worth reflecting on Rawls' challenge since in one way or another all moral matters are shaped by social organisation. Rawls' own answer (but not the only one) is this:

There should be two main principles of social justice, and the first should take precedence over the second where they conflict.

1. Each person should have an equal right to the maximum amount of liberty consistent with a similar liberty for others. In other words, each person should have as much freedom as possible unless or until this freedom works against the freedoms of other people. The basic liberties, according to Rawls, are political liberty, the right to property, freedom from arbitrary arrest, and to be within a system of law which deals impartially with all who come under its rule.
2. Any social and economic inequalities should be organised so that they work to everyone's advantage, including the worst-off. In a modern and complex society, which is bound to contain people of different abilities, there will inevitably be some inequalities. But if these work only for the benefit of those already privileged they should not be allowed. An example of a justifiable inequality, on Rawls' account, is for a surgeon to be well off, but only because his skills have the potential to contribute to the well-being of all. Societies without the services of rich surgeons will be worse off, Rawls thinks.

Like any argument in moral and political philosophy, Rawls' position is open to criticism. It has, for example, been argued that his response is by no means the only feasible conclusion that might be reached from behind the veil. Why, for instance, does Rawls prefer liberty above equality? Some people might well conclude that the best way to ensure social justice is to guarantee equal distribution of resources, even at the price of reduced personal liberty. After all, we are not asked to imagine contractors already living in a liberal social regime, but people whose political outlooks are entirely unpolluted by experience and education. Indeed, Rawls' own judgement does not appear to have been made in total ignorance, but is informed by prior adherence to liberal ideals. He assumes that the 'rational person' behind the veil of ignorance is rational in a particular way. Regardless of the actual identity of surgeons and dustmen, the ignorant rationalist is supposed to think it right *a priori* that such grossly unequal roles and status should exist in a just society.

Rawls does not expect that social structures different from those which presently make up Western society will be entertained for long. He does not envisage anyone behind the veil prepared to argue for absolute equality of education for fear he might then be at risk through the absence of trained surgeons. But of course it is by no means absurd to think that some contractors might be prepared to bargain for a system of education that does not create elite specialisms. It is not out of the question that a different system of education could eliminate the need for so many surgeons, nor is it necessarily the case that a more egalitarian system of education, and even more equal later financial reward, will result in a scarcity of trained surgeons (people might just decide to become surgeons for the challenge and job satisfaction).

The pros and cons of Rawls' theory of justice are not a major concern for this inquiry, however. But what is central is the powerful connection between politics and morality that Rawls' work highlights. The political structure of a society is intimately linked to the level of morality. If social structures enable some people to achieve worthwhile potentials but do not allow others equivalent chances – then morality is not being created as fully as it should be.

In the concluding chapters of this book it is argued that since work for health is a moral endeavour, and that since part of the purpose of health care is to act justly, then the entire performance of the health service – its administration, its hierarchies, its priorities, and its resourcing – is of moral concern because it is directly and constantly responsible for creating or diminishing the degree of morality in the world.

## SUMMARY

Chapter Seven has given an elementary account of classic approaches to moral reasoning. This, together with Chapter Five's discussion of the foundation of morality, should provide health workers with sufficient background material to begin to reflect with some confidence about morality in health care. It also serves as essential preparation for understanding and using the Ethical Grid.

# CHAPTER EIGHT

# Obstacles to Clear Moral Reasoning

Moral reasoning can be polluted by inappropriate ways of thinking. Some of these impurities – in particular 'bad faith' and health economics – are discussed in this chapter.

## BAD FAITH

Honesty and integrity are essential in moral reasoning. One way to reveal their importance is to contemplate 'bad faith'.

According to Jean-Paul Sartre, people guilty of bad faith fail to be true to themselves – they deny their individuality and freedom by burying it in a role. Unfortunately, playing out a predefined role is a characteristic commonly displayed by people who become professionals. As we have seen, when some people become 'professional' they seem to change – sometimes quite radically – from how they were before. Their very identities appear to alter to fit the position taken on. Some become so addicted they imagine 'professional moral responsibility' is different from 'personal moral responsibility', and become morally lost as a result (the soldier blindly carrying out orders, the surgeon who thinks his job is only to cut and stitch, the lawyer happy to have persuaded a jury to acquit her guilty client – each exhibits this tendency).

Sartre saw that we must all cope with an irrational world – a world, despite superficial appearances, without order and structure. In this random universe things just happen and we have no real control over them (rather like Nottingham Forest's defence strategy in recent years – sad to say). Nothing is determined. Events are free and conform to no pattern. Our canons of rationality, logic, order, and coherence are only façade. Reality is chaotic and meaningless. We categorise the world, and we categorise ourselves. We must, for if we did not we would feel permanently disorientated – forever anguished and nauseous. However by creating a comforting, artificial world we lose touch with what is truly real, and forget our true nature.

Bad faith results from habitual denial of this truth. Once we see ourselves as bound to act in a certain way, once we say, 'I have no choice in this matter' then we have deceived ourselves and are acting in bad faith. Bad faith is the failure to realise that any role has originally been a matter of choice, and that it remains a matter of choice whether to continue to perform it or not.

Bad faith is exhibited, for example, when a person buys a luxury item – perhaps a watch with a plain granite face which makes telling the time a matter of guesswork – and justifies the purchase by saying it was essential. There are many who see themselves as a stereotype – as the dutiful housewife with two children, cooking meals at set times for her husband, just as her mother did before her; or as the kindly paternalistic general practitioner; or as the angry, certain, righteous member of Militant; or as the total feminist; or as the idle erudite philosopher sponging a good wage from the State, always 'writing a book' but never finishing it. These people's tastes, beliefs, and actions are dictated not by themselves but by the roles they play.

Sartre thought that the man who exhibits bad faith is striving to become an object, sacrificing creativity for the security of a tried and trusted role. The man with bad faith tries to become an object in order to lose true consciousness, and as a result abdicates responsibility. He throws away choice for the sake of becoming a pawn. Bad faith is a personal disgrace, for where there is no real choice there can be no moral development. For Sartre, no matter what the rules, there is always choice. Not to recognise this is to ossify – which is the worst crime a person can commit against himself.

Although Sartre's philosophy may be difficult to accept – and this book certainly does not argue that health professionals should act as if the world is chaotic – his insight is illuminating and has ramifications for moral action.

## ESSENCE AND EXISTENCE – AN EXPANSION

This book's central questions are: What are human beings for? What is it about us that makes our existence truly worthwhile, and what is it that degrades us? Of course these are not matters that can be finally proved, but they should be constantly discussed.

Thus Sartre's contribution is important in two ways. First he reminds us of the presence of our remarkable capacity for free choice, and then shows that the existence of this capacity has implications for the way societies and their institutions are arranged.

Sartre drew a fundamental distinction between people and objects. Objects – chairs, satchels or beer mugs, for instance – have an essence. What they are is predetermined, their nature fixed according to their given function. But people are not like this. We do not have an allotted essence or 'shape' as objects do. People simply have existence, a fact which allows unadulterated freedom to create oneself uniquely. So much freedom is so frightening that many of us feel unable to face up to it, preferring to think of ourselves as essences instead.

Sartre's idea is as naïve as it is penetrating. It takes no account of genetics, for instance, and fails to appreciate that no one has infinite potential. Nor does it recognise how greatly people can be constrained by external circumstances and events (as Sartre was to realise later in his life). But despite these considerable oversights, Sartre's moral ideal is enormously important.

# A FURTHER PROBLEM

It is a fact of life that very many of us are content to be instructed. Not everyone wants to take responsibility, and not everyone is inclined to take creative risks. Some people insist there is much they would rather not know, even about their medical treatment. Some of us do not want autonomy (Understanding B – see p. 180) because it is taxing, and it can hurt. Most of us are trusting, submissive and happy to have our horizons defined for us. Why should people not spend their lives in cotton wool if that is what they wish? Why should people not freely decide to abdicate their autonomy in favour of being looked after by the State, an institution, or another person?

In answer, there are two reasons why personal deliberation and independent choosing should be encouraged in all forms of human life, including professional life. First, a person trained habitually to follow given rules is underdeveloped. A vital part of her is left barren when it could be verdant. In extreme cases such a person will have difficulty making any social choices coherently. Even when someone operates under a system of rules there is still need for some deliberation. Is this a situation of the kind in which I should apply this rule? In this case, is this procedure justified? Which of the rules I could use should I choose just now? Second, such a person is not properly equipped to deal with unexpected life circumstances – precisely the situations health workers often face. The rare case, the novel issue (perhaps raised by advances in medical technology), the urgent problem when there is no time to consult the rule book or a superior – all these occur repeatedly. Only someone who has developed his capacity to judge can act thoughtfully – committed rule-followers must stand helplessly by, redundant without their guide. Those who think for themselves are in an infinitely better position. They can follow rules if they believe it wise to do so, and they can override them if they think they should.

## An Illustration

It is not so difficult to imagine what it is like to throw off the shackles of bad faith. There is an enlightening illustration of the dizziness, the sense of being a stranger in a foreign land, the freedom and the fear, that people can experience when they first try to shake off their bad faith. Yet this illustration is so mundane, and the step so small.

When driving road vehicles it is the law that we must stop at traffic lights on the signal red. In order to avoid accidents and ensure the traffic flows smoothly it can – obviously – be important to obey this particular rule. Occasionally traffic lights fail and we have to make our own judgement about whether or not it is safe to proceed. So it is for the best that we can choose to disobey faulty signals if we need to. But this is not the most interesting case. Sometimes we are not sure if the traffic lights are working properly. Perhaps it is late at night, there is little traffic, and the lights seem to have been on red for a very long time. The rule-follower's car is four cars away from the front of the queue. Then, hesitantly, the leading car begins to move forward despite the red light. It moves away and, again hesitantly, the next car follows, and then the third. What is the committed rule-follower to do?

Once he decides to move it will be like a revelation. Almost magically the rules will melt away, the silly red traffic light will become metal and glass and electrics. The rules will be seen as temporary, man-made, expedient, and of minor importance. The rule is not necessary at all, even though it is usually useful. It can be superseded by human judgement. The rule-follower will have been given a glimpse of what it feels like to begin to lose bad faith.

It might be argued that bad faith is a fanciful idea. One has only to observe how many people accept so many social rules without question. Indeed, many people do not even understand that questions are possible. In Britain, for instance, most people accept that the British version of democracy is the only true democracy (despite the existence of several alternative systems around the world), that education for most children should cease at the age of sixteen, and countless other traditions too. It seems to most people that these things have always been part of British life, and so they assume there can be no other way.

However, just as the belief that things in Britain have always been more or less as they are now is false, so it is also a myth that most people can act only on pregiven rules. Anyone who employs moral reasoning properly – weighing and balancing rules, duties, and consequences in order to obtain the best possible outcome – transcends what has been given to her. And all competent people surely have this ability – it is there if we want to use it.

It is also wrong to believe that most of us are unable to recognise the absurd and transient nature of the world. Happily not everyone is an existentialist of Sartre's calibre but people do become aware of the fragility of existence, and the impermanence of even the most precious aspects of life. Because of this it is both right and practical to say: 'Here is a tool – it is not something which can give you certain answers because, as with so much in life, nothing is certain in the moral realm. But it is something which can help you use your judgement.'

None of this is provable, of course. If it is not true that people possess the ability to think for themselves – or if we are deluded when we believe we are thinking freely – then it is probably a waste of time to provide a general tool to enhance ethical deliberation. But it is at least plausible that the ability to see beyond convention and apparent order is a part of our intellectual make-up. All people, unless they die at an early age, sooner or later become aware that familiar 'certainties' can fall away. They vanish when a person is suddenly made redundant after long service, when parents divorce, and when someone close dies or leaves. These and countless other crises force the recognition that the existence we have come to feel safe with is actually acutely brittle. People with no ability to see this are extremely unusual. For instance, if a parent suffers the death of a child at Christmas then the trimmings, bonhomie and tinsel will appear alien, superficial, and unreal. If they do not – even if only temporarily – then this would concern a health worker who wished to facilitate the grieving process, and may well indicate severe psychological disorder.

# A FURTHER OBSTACLE TO CLEAR MORAL REASONING. QALYs: THE WRONG KIND OF COST-BENEFIT ANALYSIS

It is easiest to measure those things that can be measured most easily. But it is not always true that the most measurable things are the most valuable.

> It is the mark of the educated man and a proof of his culture that in every subject he looks for only so much precision as nature permits.[30]

## CAN QALYs BE A TOOL FOR A HEALTH SERVICE?

QALYs is an acronym for Quality Adjusted Life Years, and 'the QALY' a measure intended to enable the efficient calculation of health service priorities. The QALY is the most well-known tool of health economics, and embodies all that is wrong with this one-eyed approach to policy-making.[57-60] In common with other forms of consequentialism QALYs are controversial, though the nature of the controversy is not always clear because the continuing debate tends to generate different sorts of question. Different people expect – and fear – different things from QALYs. Health economists, managers with fixed budgets, doctors facing torturous choices, and moral philosophers reflecting at a safe distance, each focuses on their most familiar aspects. The economist wants to improve the QALY – so as to make it a more reliable measure; the doctor wonders whether QALYs can help her make efficient decisions; the manager wants to use them to make implicit priorities more explicit; while the philosopher worries about their morality.

## WHAT IS A QALY?

In the words of Alan Williams, one of the founders of the QALY idea:

> The essence of a QALY is that it takes a year of healthy life expectancy to be worth 1, but regards a year of unhealthy life expectancy as worth less than 1. Its precise value is lower the worse the quality of life of the unhealthy person (which is what the 'quality adjusted' bit is all about). If being dead is worth zero, it is, in principle, possible for a QALY to be negative, i.e. for the quality of a person's life to be judged worse than being dead.
>
> The general idea is that a beneficial health care activity is one that generates a positive amount of QALYs, and that an efficient health care activity is one where the cost per QALY is as low as it can be. A high priority health care activity is one where the cost-per-QALY is low, and a low priority activity is one where the cost-per-QALY is high.[61]

Practically speaking the QALY is a way to assess differences in the quality of life of different individuals. The results it produces are meant to be used in situations where resources are scarce. And it is this application – the use of the QALY to justify rationing – that causes the trouble.

Some critics argue that QALYs are an attempt to dress up discrimination against the sick, elderly and non-productive in pseudo-technical language. Amongst a lot else, they say the QALY fudges a vital distinction between *quality* of life and the *value* of life, assuming that if a life's quality decreases then its value must drop proportionately. This, it is argued, is an insidious mistake, illustrated by the following *non sequitur*:

1. More 'health output' (or more QALYs – if one accepts the crude definition of health put forward by some health economists)[57] is achieved by spending the same amount of money on Fred as on John.
2. Better cost-effectiveness is obtained by treating Fred rather than John.
3. Therefore Fred's life has more value than John's.

But the value of life is not what it costs to maintain it. If one makes an alternative distinction – between basic 'persons' and 'full persons', for example – then there are good reasons for not confusing value with cost. Although full persons have myriad talents, all people have basic capacities which imply a fundamental equality. There may be huge differences in the quality of their lives – but there can be no differences in the value of their lives seen this way. Just as the criminal law makes no distinction between the murder of a one-year old and the murder of an adult, personal existence is equally valuable whether one is 2, 15 or 90. The QALY – on the other hand – assumes the value of human life is not morally fixed but is a 'variable' that can change according to a person's age, ability, and social status.

## HOW ARE QALYs MEANT TO BE USED?

QALYs may be used for different purposes. They might be employed to decide which of a range of treatments open to a patient will bring about the most favourable quality of life – an ethically inoffensive use. Alternatively they might be used to discriminate between patients in competition for a scarce resource – an ethically troublesome use. There are other modes lying between these extremes. QALYs can be deployed in the following ways:

1. To clarify costs of treatment, without generating practical change.
2. To make priorities explicit, so encouraging more self-conscious and rigorous thinking.
3. To compare and assess treatments which produce short-term benefit against those which produce benefit in the long term.
4. To ensure the most cost-effective use of health service funds. For example, hip-replacement operations are said to be more cost-effective in QALY terminology than heart transplants. It was noted in *The Economist* that studies at York University had come to the conclusion that heart transplants cost over £5000 per QALY compared with £1000 for coronary by-passes and £750 for hip-replacements.[62] Since health service funding is finite it was concluded that it is better to channel available funds into hip-replacement operations.
5. To ensure the most beneficial distribution, in utilitarian terms, of any available scarce resource – renal dialysis or a drug in short supply, for example.

6. To select for treatment those people who might be expected to produce the most QALYs. Such selection is reminiscent of the policy used by armies which treat first of all those soldiers most likely to return quickly to the battle.
7. To make apparently reflective judgements merely a matter of calculation.

## AGAINST QALYs

Before considering objections to the use of QALYs it is important to place the current controversy in more general perspective. The debate actually represents nothing more than the swing of a pendulum between deontology and consequentialism. At present there is great emphasis on the assessment of the consequences of actions, as a gauge to their worth. But this fashion – and it is nothing more – misses so much of importance in human life, and misses it so blatantly, that it will not last for long: cutting costs is a pointless exercise if it is done only for its own sake.

Sooner or later any form of utilitarianism becomes absurd if it is not part of a wider picture. For example, Jeremy Bentham invented the Felicific Calculus, meant to help people decide what to do, based on an assessment of likely consequences (roughly, the more pleasure an action is likely to produce the more reason to do it). Bentham took into account the type, intensity and duration of pleasure, and argued for a standard scale by which to calculate. His hope was that everyone would agree on this standard. But, just like QALYs, his strategy was doomed to failure because different people have different ideas about how to rate pleasures. Imagine, for illustration, how difficult it would be for any group of people from dissimilar backgrounds to agree about the relative merits of reading a good novel, eating a large bar of chocolate, getting drunk with friends on Saturday night, robbing a bank, or whatever other entertainment is proposed.

In defence of the Felicific Calculus it should be said that Bentham took other people's pleasures into account, arguing that the worth of human actions should be seen against a background of pleasure generated overall. However, just as they share the inability to settle on objective measures, in application both Bentham's Calculus and QALYs flounder ethically because they can legitimise extravagant discrimination. So long as the general balance is more 'good' than 'bad' then actions – whatever they are – are said to be justified (for Bentham the 'good' is pleasure and the 'bad' pain, while for the advocates of QALYs life protected cheaply is 'good' while expensive life is 'bad').

Both ways of calculation are deeply contrary to justice as fairness. It is worth recalling an illustration to emphasise the point. If we are given the option of having a disease-free, war-free, content, and wholly productive society at the single cost of knowing that one human being will be kept in eternal and perpetual agony of mind and body, should we accept? If they are honest, consequentialists (and therefore almost all economists) have to agree to the contract – or else relinquish all consistency – yet the injustice of the situation is obvious.

The following specific points may be made against QALYs:

## I.  Their Content is Arbitrary

QALY criteria – degree of pain, length of expected life, and degree of disability – are at worst arbitrary and at best governed by a health service preoccupied with economics, mortality, and morbidity. In the absence of a theory of health service purpose there is no reason why these components should have been chosen before, for example, intelligence, amount of past income, amount of body hair, height, or eye colour. Why not these measures? If a person is unfortunate enough to be completely bald, quite small, rather stupid, and to have been unemployed for a long time it might be concluded that her quality of life is low, and that someone else ought to be treated in her stead.

These criteria would quickly be condemned as unfair and arbitrary – discriminating solely according to a person's bad luck – but of course this is precisely what the QALY measure does. The criteria might sound more objective, gaining credibility from the traditional medical context, but they have been selected from an indefinite range of alternatives. If you are old or disabled or in pain or immobile – tough luck. It does not matter that you devote your life to charity – you are 78 and not worth as much as the 25-year-old business man with two children.

## 2.  QALYs Impose Subjective Values on Other Subjects (and claim objectivity as they do so)[60]

Their use to discriminate between people means that arbitrary or biased criteria are imposed on those who do not share their way of thinking. Worse still, many economists[63] claim their advice is unbiased, or value-neutral, when this is patently not the case.

## 3.  QALYs Promote Many Myths

Among them:

a. That it is possible to be certain about the outcomes of treatment, that we know how long people will live, that my pain is the same as your pain, and that the QALY caiculation can be carried out without difficulty and without assumptions.
b. That in all cases where QALYs are used to discriminate it is feasible to calculate what to do. The idea that each human being is unique, and that each of us has defining qualities that cannot be measured, is not considered. Just as only a partial aspect of moral reasoning is recognised, it is assumed that all health service cases are, by and large, governed by the same few factors (see Palmer[64] for a perfect example of this blinkered view).

The selection of 'easy' cases as examples helps further this latter myth. For instance, if the choice lies between offering scarce life-saving treatment to a 35-year-old man with a good career and a young family, or to help a 70-year old with no close relatives then – all else being equal – QALYs explain why it makes sense to discriminate against the older man. But it is a different matter if the choice is between a 13-year-old boy and an 11-year-old girl. If only one can be treated and the primary discriminatory measures – length of expected life and treatment cost – are not applicable, and all other selected criteria are equal, then the QALY is no help at all. The reason why it is morally difficult to discriminate between two children is that we have a deep feeling they are entitled to equal respect and so equal treatment. And the feeling remains in the case of the 35-year old and the 70-year old – why are these two people not entitled to equal respect if the boy and girl are?

## 4.  The Slippery Slope

It should by now be obvious how easily the acceptance of QALYs makes it to slide down a slope where injustice to some can be 'justified' as being in the interest of the majority. This is the justification Hitler used to explain the murder of Jews – it was said to be in the interest of the German nation as a whole – and lies behind apartheid and the two great twentieth-century dictatorships (in Russia and China).

QALYs inevitably discriminate on the ground of age, and can readily be used to discriminate on grounds of race, sex, or class. If you are old then your life expectancy is usually less than if you are young, so if there is to be a straight choice between the old and the young the old must be sacrificed, regardless of how much they want to live, how much they have to give, or how much they value their futures.

If you are a woman your life expectancy is longer than a man's, therefore you should receive the scarce resource – all other things being equal. But if you are a woman you might suffer from some medical conditions men do not. If the treatment for these is more expensive than the treatment for his, and there is not enough money to go round, then you might find that you will not be treated yet he will.

Epidemiological studies inform us that different races suffer from different diseases and have different life expectancies. So do the different classes. A member of parliament can expect a longer life than a mineworker so again, all other things being equal, the MP should be treated at the expense of the mineworker.

It does not require a massive leap of imagination to understand how QALYs could be used to justify non-voluntary euthanasia, or allowing handicapped infants to die, or the abandonment of mental patients of no danger to society. Defenders of QALYs might argue that safeguards could be built into the system, and already exist in most Western legislation, but if that is so reassuring why not pick a better system in the first place?

## THE BENEFIT OF QALYs

The main benefit of open discussion about QALYs is that they expose the implicit, though often unintentional and unavoidable, injustice of some decisions taken in the present health service – injustice which might be avoided given different structure and funding. QALYs remind us that health service resources are usually scarce not as a result of nature but as a consequence of a human decision to spend money elsewhere, for instance on weapons of war, on luxuries, on fast cars, on houses with more rooms than we need, and so on. Spending on weapons, for instance, is usually 'justified' on the ground that they act to preserve human life, by deterring warmongers. But the preservation of human life is a central role for medical services too, and in a more direct and continuous sense. Since war is not imminent there is surely a case (which bad faith tends to obscure) that at least some military defence money be transferred to medical services constantly involved in the defence of human life.

# WHAT SHOULD BE DONE?

John Harris has proposed that the only fair way to distribute a scarce resource is to draw lots. If, for instance, there are ten potential patients and only one bed available in an intensive care unit then clinical circumstances should not be taken into account, rather the decision should be left to chance. The patient who draws the longest straw should be helped – even if she stands less chance of a good recovery than her fellow gamblers. This is fair in the sense that everyone has an equal chance, but is it practicable? Would any doctor ever carry out such a lottery? It seems unlikely, not least because the doctor would almost certainly face legal action if she did.

So we are left with two unacceptable alternatives: to discriminate between people as a matter of policy – thus offending a basic principle of civilised society that all people are entitled to equal respect, regardless of their luck or their talents – or to be undiscriminating, drawing lots for a scant resource. But this seems neither practical nor cost-effective. Randomness by itself does not amount to a policy of equal respect. How could a doctor explain to a mother that her young child had been sacrificed as the result of a lottery, to save an old man with only months left to live?

## WHAT IS NEEDED IS EXPERIENCE, CONSIDERATION, AND THE ABILITY TO REASON MORALLY

Sometimes hard choices have to be faced. Where decisions have to be made about who to treat and who not to treat doctors need guidance. It is not entirely immoral to treat the 15-year old rather than the 95-year old, or the 25-year old with a minor illness rather than the terminally ill 25-year old, but in order to show this a complete deliberation is necessary – not just an economic one.

Because each situation is unique the idea of applying a crude quantitative measure only is unsuitable. What is worse, the use of QALYs might turn doctors into calculating machines where they come to believe that moral judgements are a matter of measuring simple differences. Once this has become habit doctors might begin to think that computed answers are not their responsibility but somehow objective, disregarding the fact they have chosen to use the measure in the first place. What is needed is not an unjust technique but responsible, caring individuals and organisations – humane systems, not purely economic ones.

### Two Practical Proposals

1. That education in moral reasoning be given to all medical practitioners and health workers, on a regular basis. Health workers should be given education in analysis of

interventions, in weighing up strengths and weaknesses of alternatives, in the use of logic, in law, and in the assessment of duties and consequences.

It should be explained that ethics is a process of deliberation in which it is necessary to select certain priorities from a range of possibilities. In any ethical deliberation in health work four levels should be addressed: external considerations such as evidence for one's judgement, duties, consequences, and the core rationale of health work. Once this core is understood health workers will know that the unqualified use of QALYs is not proper work for health. Their use may create autonomy in some individuals, respect the autonomy of some individuals, and will serve some needs before wants (and some wants before needs) but the use of QALYs cannot be said to treat people with equal respect.

2. That since 'scarce resources' are scarce only as a result of lack of funds that might be available from other sources, and since by the use of statistics it is possible to predict fairly accurately how many dialysis machines and other such resources will be needed, it should become public knowledge that lives are being lost and those doctors who must decide are being placed in impossible positions as a result of human priorities, not natural circumstances.

Consequently whenever a health worker has to make a 'tragic choice' – sacrificing a life where that life could have been saved – there should be a recognised professional facility for this to be publicly recorded. This could be done through Medical Associations, who could ensure accuracy, and publicised each month in national newspapers. Since newspapers regularly print stories of murder and road death as examples of avoidable injustice this should not be unappealing to them. It might even be desirable to have a league table of 'enforced injustice in medicine'.

In this way QALYs can work for good. If the measure ever does have to be used it should not be used on its own, without also considering justice and unintended consequences, for instance. And it should not be seen as an objective rule. But if, in the hard world of medicine and health, the QALY measure does have to be a part of an assessment it should never be used in such a way as to legitimise discrimination, as if it is the only possible choice, as if it is the only moral choice, or as if it ought to be part of a true system of health care. It is not the only alternative and should not be used exclusively.

## CONCLUSION

This chapter has outlined obstacles in the path of clear moral reasoning. Such obstacles should be avoided by health workers. If they are not overcome it is impossible to use the Ethical Grid properly.

# How to Make Ethically Sound Practical Decisions

# CHAPTER NINE

# The Rings of Uncertainty

Part Three offers a set of ethically based decision-making devices to health workers. The most important of these is the Ethical Grid.

This chapter explains the Rings of Uncertainty – a preliminary decision-making device. Though originally intended to offer analytic guidance to morally motivated doctors[10] the Rings can be employed by any health worker. They may be used in conjunction with the Ethical Grid, and are particularly effective when outlining pros and cons and establishing a mental picture to expose to ethical scrutiny.

## INTRODUCTION

Given that health professionals often wish to work for health in a sense which goes beyond work against disease, how might they assess their most appropriate roles? How might they decide when not to intervene, or when they should cease? This chapter suggests a way for health workers to picture their positions in a world of uncertainty. By means of this picturing they will be better placed to judge the most desirable courses to steer.

'What role ought a health worker adopt?' 'What should limit her activity?' At the moment health workers are guided primarily by precedent and subjective judgement. Apart from the Ethical Grid (which has not yet been universally adopted) there is no substantial framework to help a health worker arrive at a systematically reasoned position. As a result it is often difficult for other health workers – doctors, nurses, managers and patients – to challenge the reasoning processes which led to an intervention. The vague phrase 'I exercised my clinical/nursing/managerial judgement' is still used to conceal woolly or dubious thinking – and other health professionals do not possess a mutual structure to enable encouragement or restraint. If a nurse thinks a doctor is not doing enough to help a patient, or a manager believes a nurse is going too far, there is no shared, logical means by which to facilitate discussion. Consequently confrontation regularly occurs where constructive conversation might have taken place.

By presenting a graphic, graspable model for health workers to reflect upon possible roles and interventions, this chapter attempts to increase understanding of the philosophical basis of health work. It also suggests a means of enhancing communication between health workers of all kinds – to the benefit of those for whom they care.

The framework is not meant to be dogmatic but to support health workers' deliberations. Many health care decisions fall within the province of personal judgement. Furthermore, there is rarely only one answer to a problem. Usually there are alternative possibilities, each of which has merit. However, there are limits which distinguish acceptable answers from the unacceptable. The Rings of Uncertainty and the Autonomy Test (explained in Chapter Ten) are designed to reveal clear boundaries beyond which health workers ought not to act, although they should have a high degree of liberty within them.

## THE RINGS OF UNCERTAINTY

The Rings can best be explained in a series of steps.

### STEP ONE

Represented generally in Figure 11, uncertainty is the most abiding and pervasive limit on health work.

The traditional aim of health work is to move from the outside to the inside – to come ever closer to certainty. However, when this abstract idea is specifically expressed it can be seen that inward progress is not necessarily the most appropriate direction. It is sometimes better that a doctor (for instance) moves outwards in the Rings – especially if she thinks of herself as a general problem-solver who wants to work for health.

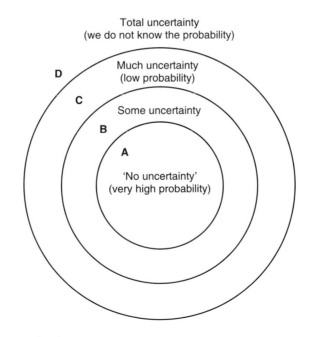

**Figure 11**   The Rings in the abstract

Although this may not be the safest option – it becomes more likely she will be exposed to criticism – there are considerable benefits to be had. For example, by stretching outwards a doctor might learn from other people and so extend her competence, she might discover fresh and broader options for problem-solving, new approaches and methods might become apparent and – perhaps most important of all – by welcoming the idea of outward travel rather than constantly seeking shelter in certainty, her flexibility may increase. She may learn when to be humble and when it is best to be passive. Indeed it is only by facing outwards as well as in that anyone can work for health in the richest sense.[65]

The basic diagram can be adapted to show each limit to health work. Consider first the Rings expressed for technical competence.

## STEP TWO: THE RINGS EXPRESSED

### Technical Competence

Technical competence includes both knowledge and skill. Competence (or lack of it) comes in many guises. Figure 12 translates the idea into a form suitable for the Rings of Uncertainty.

As with any general framework, the words used to describe each Ring can mean different things in different circumstances. For instance, the competencies in question might be competencies of technique, insight, or recall of information. When the Rings are expressed for resources these might be human organs, money, beds, time, or skilled people – whatever might legitimately be considered a resource. Reality must give meaning to each Ring.

Figure 12 is a simple representation of one way in which nursing activity (for instance) might be limited by competence. It is better not to imagine a nurse jumping from one section of the Rings to another. Although the Rings as illustrated appear sharply divided, in reality different levels of competence shade into each other, just as a bold scarlet can fade slowly to the palest pink. The Rings are meant to convey a steady weakening of certainty – a weakening of competence in the present case – as the nurse moves towards the outer edge.

Different sorts of question are likely to arise dependent upon the nurse's perceived position. For example, is the nurse the only person in a position to offer help? Should she intervene only with the advice and assistance of others? Is the nurse's ability to help so limited that any intervention is ill-advised?

---

**A nurse within the Rings: a practical example with reference to technical competence**

Imagine how Sally Smith might use the Rings. Sally is a nurse who has established a relationship with John Jones, a cancer patient who also suffers from moderate depression. Sally has used the Rings before and is able to picture herself actually and potentially within them. She knows that by thinking graphically she is sometimes able to reason more concretely. By using

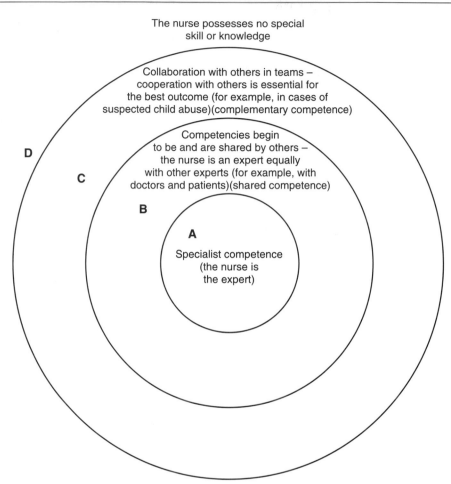

**Figure 12**   The Rings expressed for technical competence

the Rings Sally can say 'if I do that, then I shall be standing in this position within the Rings of Uncertainty'. In one sense this is to do no more than say 'if I do this, X will happen', but Sally has discovered that reference to the image can deepen her thought process.

John – a bachelor of 31 – has cancer of the bone. His doctors advise that an operation now would give him a 50% chance of a cure, but they will have to amputate his arm below the left elbow. John was distraught to learn this. To lose a limb has always been one of his biggest dreads, and to make matters worse he makes his living playing the guitar.

John refused to consent to the operation and was told that any other treatment was probably useless. In shock he informs Sally that he wishes to discharge himself from hospital.

Sally has an ethical problem to deal with, of course. However, in order to decide what to do she needs more than ethical theory, and perhaps more insight than she can obtain from independent use of the Grid. She really needs to work out where she stands in this situation, and thinks the Rings might help.

She considers the Rings expressed for competence, as shown in Figure 12. Where does she see herself? She is in the outer Rings for medical knowledge, though she is by no means a novice in oncology. But she does not have *special* knowledge, and to do anything clinical for John she would clearly have to work with a team. However, she has specialised in counselling and communication, and is the most qualified person in the department in this respect. She also knows John better than anyone else – she is a similar age and they have had several chats over the last couple of days.

If she had been a poor communicator – and had pictured herself standing at the edges of the Rings expressed for competence in this regard – she would probably have been best advised to let John leave, or to refer him on. However, not only is she in the centre Ring but the doctors have little interest in John now – they think he has made a bad decision but they cannot and will not do anything without his consent – and they have compliant patients to assist.

She resolves to set time aside to talk with John, to help him think his decision through. He agrees to this, and says he will wait in hospital until the end of her shift. As she talks with him he tells her he cannot live as a freak and cannot imagine how he will survive without his music. Sally calmly puts an opposite view and – with John's permission – introduces him to two amputees, who visit people like John. They too are in the middle of this set of Rings in these circumstances.

Unfortunately, Sally's strategy does not have the hoped-for effect. John breaks down in extreme distress. He cries and begins to rage loudly against his ill-fortune – he accuses the medics of maltreating him. At this Sally realises she is no longer in the middle Ring. At best she is at B, in a situation where other people are equally as expert as she, and she may well be at C. Knowing this she holds John, and manages to comfort and soothe him. He says he will wait on the ward while she goes to see what can be done.

Sally calls a psychiatrist and another nurse counsellor from elsewhere in the hospital. She returns to John, who agrees to see them – and the situation moves on. If it is to be resolved it will require multi-disciplinary effort and clear ethical reasoning – in fact it is now time for Sally, her colleagues and John to employ the Ethical Grid. Yet the Rings have been crucial in the early stages – without them Sally may not have felt it appropriate to intervene without the permission of her clinical colleagues, and there would now be less chance of helping John deal with his crisis.

## Other Expressions

The general Rings (Figure 11) – stretching from a core where confidence can be at a peak to a surrounding area where there is no ground for professional intervention – can be translated into several other categories. Health workers are free to suggest their own if they find the Rings helpful, or they may prefer to choose from the following selection.

## Resources

*Broader Picturing: Resources Plus Technical Competence*

The following brief example shows how complexity can begin to deepen. Envisage Dr Smith, a consultant surgeon, standing within the Rings of Uncertainty expressed for

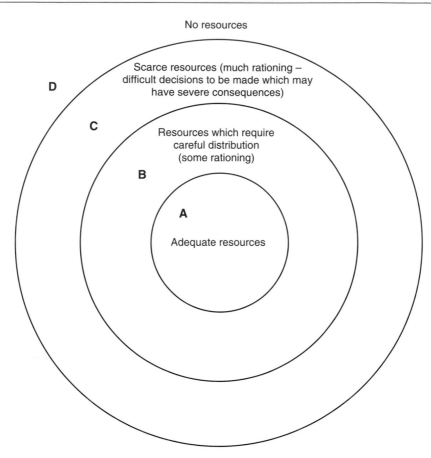

**Figure 13**    The Rings expressed for resources

resources (Figure 13). In order to work to greatest effect, to direct his time and energy along the most profitable channels, he must understand his position accurately within the Rings expressed like this. Where he can stand will depend on the extent of the resources available, and might also change according to his interpretation of the word 'resource'.

In order to arrive at the best practical approach Dr Smith should try to see himself standing simultaneously within other expressions of the Rings of Uncertainty: as if two or more Rings were superimposed one on another. For instance, if he would like to perform a heart transplant it is certain there will be resource issues. But inevitably there will be other variables to consider, of which technical competence will be one.

As far as resources are concerned, if a suitable donor organ cannot be obtained Dr Smith will be stranded in the area surrounding the Rings (D). If a compatible heart does become available then the doctor will either be operating within the outer circle (C) (where the heart is a scarce resource, and where he may have to decide who will be given it) or, if there is only one patient awaiting an organ, he will be operating within the centre Ring (A), with adequate resources in this sense at least. In this respect Dr Smith's position within the Rings is entirely subject to prevailing circumstances.

Perhaps Dr Smith wishes to transplant a kidney, has an adequate supply in his locality, but does not have sufficient funding from his health authority or hospital to pay for support staff to provide a full service. And as a consequence patients are suffering, and in some cases dying, where they need not. In this case then he is actually standing in either (C) (much rationing) or (B) (some rationing) Rings, but will almost certainly be seeking to stand within the centre Ring (A) (adequate resources).

If he wishes to make progress – if he wishes to be creative with the various limits in which he finds himself – then Dr Smith may have to consider the extent of his role within limits other than resources. For instance, if he wishes to change the situation he may have to ponder where he stands within the Rings expressed for competence, and work out where he might move within these Rings.

At present he is a single consultant lacking staff. With the advantage of his professional status he can put some pressure on hospital management, but cannot be confident he will win his way. He may have to move out from the centre to the second or third Rings – perhaps to the third Ring – where he must work in a team with other consultants, or with other health workers. If he really wants to do something in these circumstances then Dr Smith must imagine himself standing within two sets of Rings at once, and must consider where he should stand for the best within both.

## Law

Health care is a complex and uncertain affair. Given this, and given that change to a simpler system is not foreseeable, the prudent health worker will seek to recognise his position in the Rings expressed for law (Figure 14) – for he may wish to alter his practice dependent upon his perceived position. For example, he may choose to practice 'defensive medicine/nursing',[66] and so be ultracautious whenever he pictures himself in the third Ring (C), where the law is unpredictable.

The effect picturing can have on practice is not unique to the Rings expressed for law. For instance, when the Rings are expressed for technical competence a health worker may decide to be decisively in charge (perhaps when a patient sincerely asks him to do so, when a patient is very ill or unconscious, or deeply frightened) or clearly an agent for his patient, respecting the patient's beliefs and choices entirely. The health worker need not always do what a patient wants – though he must always seek to create autonomy.

## Within the Rings Expressed for Law

How should a nurse conceive of herself and her activity? And how might such picturing affect her actions? How might this help define a limit around what she might do?

Consider Emma Halsall, a practice nurse encouraged by her Health Centre to carry out simple surgical techniques, rather than refer patients on for more expensive treatment. Where should she place himself within the Rings expressed for law when a patient asks her to remove a verruca from her foot?

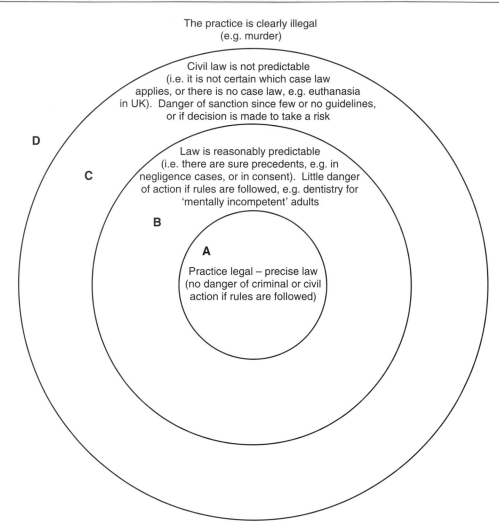

**Figure 14**    The Rings expressed for law

Should Emma picture herself in the centre Ring (A) (where the law is clear) or in another? If she thinks of herself as standing in the centre, by implication she believes she need worry only about gaining the patient's consent for the operation, so as not to risk an accusation of battery. Given this, so long as she lives up to the standard set by the Bolam Test[67] (if she is in England and Wales) she need not reflect further – particularly if she also sees herself standing within the centre of the Rings expressed for technical competence and communication. But would Emma not be wise at least to picture herself within the second Ring (B), where she chances some danger of litigation if things go wrong? If she does so she might then take great care that the operated area does not become infected, perhaps to the extent that she asks the patient back daily to check the wound. Of course, in order to decide this question, she will need to picture herself within Rings expressed for other contents, particularly technical competence and resources.

### Tension Between Different Rings

Since the Rings merely reflect considerations which must be taken into account in real-life decision-making it is often the case that, although a health worker may wish to place himself at certain points within Rings expressed for different contents, he will not be able to stand where he wants simultaneously in each Ring. Health workers can wish to move in different directions at once, and there can be irreconcilable tensions between desired positions within the Rings in some situations.

Take the case of Dr Greaves, who is consulted by a 57-year-old, retired, heavy smoking, 4 stone overweight bus-driver with a history of angina, who says that he has had to stop and sit down for 15 minutes whilst walking because he was so short of breath, and felt some pain in his chest. Should Dr Greaves decide to sit plumb in the centre of the Rings expressed for law and examine the man thoroughly, before referring him to the appropriate hospital consultant – or to Casualty – in order to attempt to prevent a possible heart attack? If he does this then he will be extremely prudent, but he will also use up valuable time. Alternatively, should Dr Greaves place himself at the centre of the Rings expressed for resources, taking care to ensure he has adequate time for each of his patients, whilst accepting the risk involved with a move into the third Ring (C) of the Rings expressed for law? If he decides to stand in (C) Ring, if he decides to send the bus-driver away after a cursory examination, then he will have placed himself in danger of an accusation of negligence – of not meeting the accepted standard of care of the competent general practitioner. What if the bus-driver actually suffers a heart attack?

## Communication

The breadth of existing language, both general and technical, will inescapably limit the extent of communication between health workers, and between health workers and patients. The study of language and communication is a complex subject.[68] The aspect of most concern to health professionals is usually the extent to which meaning is understood: does the patient/client have a clear picture of what I have said? Have I properly grasped what the patient is trying to describe to me?

Consider pain. Pain can be an intensely meaningful word, but is notoriously difficult to translate accurately. When a person is asked if she feels pain she is commonly asked for its location and severity, and most of us can relate this. But if more detail is needed it is difficult, if not impossible, to tell whether intended meaning has been correctly conveyed. If she explains that the pain is 'stabbing' or 'deep' or 'intense' this may not be enough to establish a clear clinical picture without further investigation. And even if it is sufficient for a clinical assessment, it may nonetheless not put across a faithful representation of the pain. If a more detailed and extensive 'pain language' could be devised and made common currency then the limits of language might stretch to allow more extensive communication.

There are other examples of the way the limit on what may be communicated can expand. For instance, the language of psychiatry develops regularly.[69] And as new technology is invented (for example, 'body scanning' by 'magnetic resonance' or 'genetic engineering') so new words and uses of language become necessary to describe the images produced. Equally, the limits may shrink. Some commentators[70] have argued that this process occurred in the 1960s when 'reductionist science' enjoyed its heyday. (Reductionism is the belief that the way to understand more about nature is to gain knowledge about ever smaller parts of it. Thus it might be held that more can be learnt about disease through biochemistry than through social research.) During this era words and phrases such as 'holistic', 'spiritual healing' and 'person-centred' were considered empty by many scientists.

Figure 15 suggests one way of representing levels of communication using the Rings of Uncertainty. The wording implies language in the sense of shared meaning between those who wish to communicate.

This is only one possible formulation of the Rings expressed for language and communication. The simple model cannot, without overstretching credibility and coherence, accommodate all possibilities. It is one simple image of communication among the many which can be found in work in the philosophy of language. No attempt is made here to deal with its philosophical difficulties – for instance, how does one actually check whether idea (1) remains idea (1) or has become idea (3)? However, it will suffice for the most familiar difficulties of language use. It is not uncommon to underestimate the extent of these, and the levels of language and communication are therefore an important inclusion.

For example, whether using technical or common language, it is often not clear that full comprehension has occurred. It is well known that the use of technical terms without explanation can generate confusion. As we have seen, 'ethics' has a variety of meanings. For some 'ethics' means 'a personal code of behaviour' and for others 'rules governing society'. And while 'therapy' may be a neutral or enabling activity for most therapists, for some patients the word can carry connotations of blame and punishment. Some patients assume they are responsible for their illness, and see therapy as a form of penance – 'I would not need therapy had I been a better person.' If what is meant is not specified clearly then misunderstanding is likely.

Misunderstandings can occur as the result of under-elaboration (for example, 'go to bed and take bed-rest' might imply a day or a week of confinement); misperception of emphasis (for example, 'this operation has some risk, like all operations' might mean one thing to the doctor and quite another to the patient, not least because it is the patient who must undergo the operation and the doctor who must perform or observe it); and misinterpretation through ambiguity (for example, the words 'safe', 'cancer' and 'love' have a range of meanings). A good health worker must be careful that comprehension is as accurate as possible. It can be a valuable exercise for a health worker habitually to attempt to picture herself within the Rings expressed this way.

Although the Rings are not intended for urgent situations it can be helpful to have them in mind during some consultations. In especially fraught meetings the level of understanding can quickly change. Some news can have a dramatic effect on communication. To take one example, in a discussion between a doctor and patient

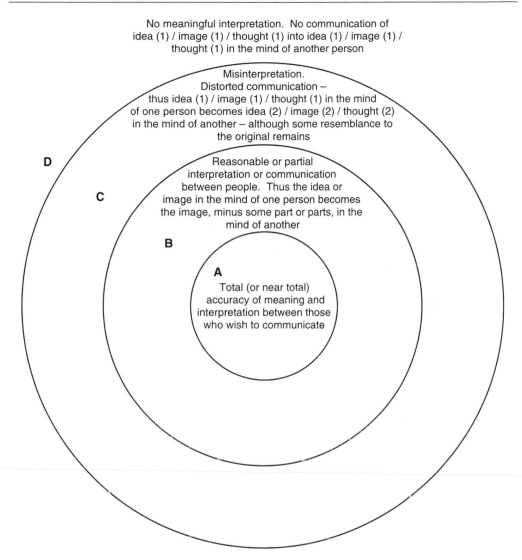

No meaningful interpretation.  No communication of
idea (1) / image (1) / thought (1) into idea (1) / image (1) /
thought (1) in the mind of another person

Misinterpretation.
Distorted communication –
thus idea (1) / image (1) / thought (1) in the mind
of one person becomes idea (2) / image (2) / thought (2)
in the mind of another – although some resemblance to
the original remains

Reasonable or partial
interpretation or communication
between people.  Thus the idea or
image in the mind of one person becomes
the image, minus some part or parts, in the
mind of another

A
Total (or near total)
accuracy of meaning and
interpretation between those
who wish to communicate

D

C

B

**Figure 15**    The Rings expressed for communication

from similar backgrounds (both professionals, both white, both men, both middle
class, and both in their fifties) about the results of exploratory tests, communication
may take place within either Rings (A) or (B), until a certain point in the conversation.
Having explained the background to the tests, and having imparted some key factual
information about the test process, when the doctor announces 'I'm afraid the results
show that you have an advanced malignancy – I'm sorry Jeff, you have cancer', the
consultation leaps to levels (C) or (D). Both the doctor and patient now inhabit an area
of heightened uncertainty.

While a person is shocked any communication is likely to be less meaningful. The
Rings can be a reminder of the need to adapt one's work to a new set of circumstances.

In addition, the fact that the level of communication has changed may affect the position of the doctor or health worker within the Rings expressed in other ways. For example, movement may be necessary within Rings expressed for resources, since more time may be required. Similarly, because shock can adversely affect the reasoning process, a fresh positioning within the Rings expressed for law and ethics might be necessary if a question of informed consent arises. If there is a serious problem of communication it may be that the Rings expressed in these ways assume the highest significance – if only temporarily.

It is now possible for a health worker who wishes to gain a clearer insight into the limits of his role to picture himself standing within the Rings of Uncertainty expressed for competence, resources, law and communication. Intriguingly, he might see himself standing at a different level for each expression of the Rings, and might notice pulls and tensions if his imagination runs contrary to reality.

But although the Rings are potentially illuminating, the model is getting confused. Simplification and more exact guidance is required. However, before this, notice that a crucial difference becomes apparent when the Rings are expressed for ethics. Whereas it is possible to offer acceptable, albeit simplistic, terminology to express the Rings in other ways, it is difficult if not impossible for ethics.

## Ethics

Two immediate difficulties are encountered when attempting to express the Rings for ethics (Figure 16). Firstly, the labels appear so open to interpretation they seem to cover many different interventions. Secondly, where one person chooses to imagine himself standing may not be the place another person would put him for the same intervention. And there seems no definite way to resolve such a disagreement.

Consider Dr White, a general practitioner, who is wondering what advice (or device) to offer Joanne who has come to see him with a request for a prescription for the contraceptive pill.

Joanne is just 15. She is categorised by those who find such classification useful as lower working class, and has a strong accent and use of English peculiar to her locality. Dr White sees he has an ethical problem. He also appreciates that he could usefully visualise himself as standing within the Rings of Uncertainty translated in other ways. For example, he might choose to express them for language and communication. Alternatively he might choose to express the Rings for law – focusing on the legal controversy which surrounded the Gillick case[71,72] in the 1980s. However, Dr White decides that on balance his best option is to imagine himself standing within the Rings expressed for ethics.

The doctor has not been confronted with a case like this before, but is inclined towards any policy which helps other people and respects their wishes. Consequently, as Joanne begins to blurt out she wants the Pill, his basic instinct is to talk it through with her and then, all being well, to prescribe the most appropriate drug. Dr White decides to clarify his position – because he knows his instinct is not shared by all doctors, and suspects it might be important to analyse the situation. But, as he conjures up his mental picture of a series of rings and tries to see himself within them, the image is

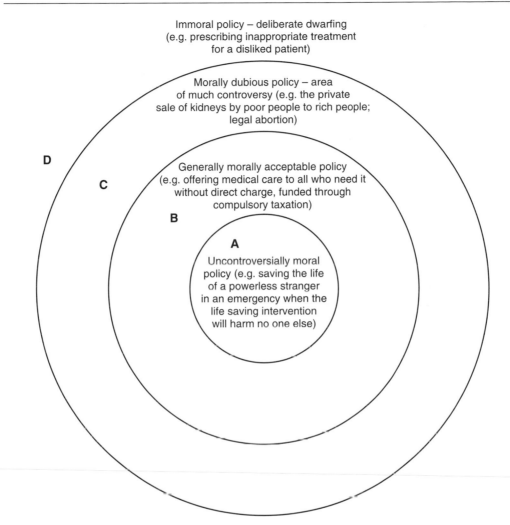

**Figure 16**  The Rings expressed for ethics

muddled. He can see himself (and can imagine others placing him) within more than one circle.

Dr White is unsure whether to imagine himself in the second or third rings, and he is further aware that there are those who would argue – vehemently in some cases – that by considering prescribing an oral contraceptive to a sexually active girl under the age of consent he is standing in area (D) (Mrs Gillick took this line). He also recognises that there are some who would say he is standing in Circle (A) (people in the Women's Rights Movement usually take this view).

There is a peculiarity when the Rings are expressed for ethics: it is unlikely there will be consensus about the correct position for Dr White within the ethics Rings, yet if the Rings are expressed for law or resources controversy does not persist. In these cases Dr White's position will be open to empirical verification. The current law is that doctors

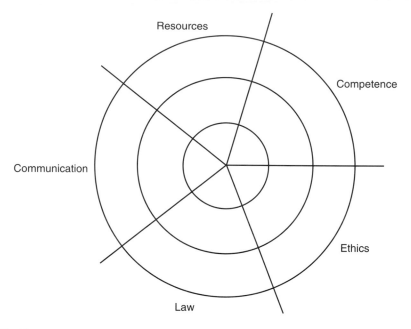

**Figure 17**  The various expressions united

can prescribe the pill to under-age girls of sufficient maturity, though they must make efforts to encourage each girl to inform her parents or guardians.[73] And there are adequate supplies of the pill, so no resource problem in this case.

As we have seen throughout this book, ethics always involves value judgements and is therefore not easy to represent in the Rings image. Ethics pervades health work, so an accurate representation would somehow show ethics saturating the Rings – since health work is a moral endeavour any application of the Rings requires ethical reflection. However, for practical reasons it is better to show ethics as a segment of the analytic process. So long as the reasoner knows this the Rings can be used to good pragmatic effect.

## The Limits of Health Work – From Insight to Guidance

It is too much to expect a health worker to retain five (or possibly more) Rings in her mind, and then to judge accurately what her role ought to be. The model needs further development.

## STEP THREE

It is possible to simplify the Rings of Uncertainty by making use of only one set of Rings divided into various segments (Figure 17).

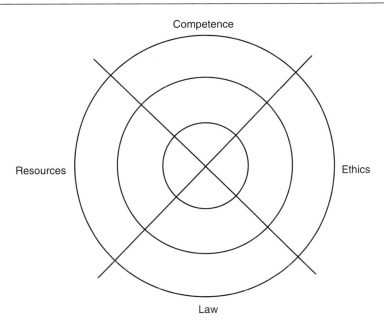

**Figure 18**    One possible set-up

## STEP FOUR

Making use of the single set of Rings, it is suggested that during the process of conceiving – during the process of picturing his position – a health worker experiments, placing markers in what he considers the appropriate sections of the segmented rings. He may decide he does not require every segment during this process. It may be that for a particular problem, a health worker thinks the main considerations are resources, competence, law and ethics, and so chooses to divide the Rings as illustrated (Figure 18).

Perhaps the doctor is a general practitioner who has to decide whether to perform a minor operation. On thinking about it, using one segmented Ring with markers, he may come up with an image like Figure 19.

This image depicts the doctor's decision. In order to arrive at it, the doctor had to consider each category. He decided he has adequate resources – he has the correct equipment, time and staff support. But where technical competence is concerned he must collaborate with others – he needs detailed advice from a consultant surgeon colleague. Ethically he thinks the policy is dubious. He worries it is a potentially risky form of cost-cutting, and that a better result might be achieved in a hospital. He also fears litigation, primarily because of his position within the technical competence segment.

On balance the GP decides not to do it. But his decision was imprecise. It would be possible, but very cumbersome, to translate the decision-making process into a series of hypotheses and tests. A doctor might begin by forming the hypothesis, *If I operate in*

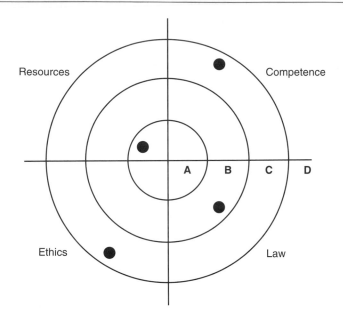

**Figure 19**    A segmented Ring with markers

*my surgery, I run no extraordinary risk.* He might then express the possible risks in terms of the categories he has selected, and assess these separately, perhaps arriving at different conclusions for law and ethics. At a later point he might test the hypothesis, *By seeking the advice of a specialist surgeon, I minimise the risk of litigation if the operation is not a success.* But this would be only one among many hypotheses he would need to test.

Naturally such exhaustive hypothesis generation and testing is rarely if ever undertaken in the clinical context. Judging and reasoning is a more fluid and agile human process than this. Fortunately, however, it is possible to add further precision to the Rings.

## STEP FIVE

### A Key Dictum

It should be obvious to all health workers that if introspection shows them standing outside the Rings of Uncertainty they ought not to intervene. This is a clear practical limit to health work. If the potential intervention appears immoral, illegal, and beyond communication, and the worker has no resources and is incompetent, then only a fool would do it. Indeed, if the health worker thinks she is outside the Rings for any segment it is doubtful she should act.

It is possible to derive a key dictum from this that *if a health worker's imagination shows him standing outside the Rings for any segment then this is a very strong indication that a limit to health work has been reached*. Unless the circumstances are exceptional, the worker should not proceed.

However, there may be exceptional circumstances. It may be that for some segments at least, to stand beyond the Rings will not necessarily require the abandonment of the project. For instance, just because an action is illegal it is not always out of the question, especially if the doctor is simultaneously standing within the Rings expressed for ethics. In some people's eyes euthanasia is a perfect example of this.

As a general guide it can be said that the further towards the edges of the Rings a health worker sees herself standing, the more reason she has to question the wisdom of her situation or plan. But this guideline is still too general to be of much practical use. What if the health worker has divided her Ring of Uncertainty into four segments and conceives of herself as standing in the centre for two and at the edges of the outer ring for the other two segments? How is she to assess her most appropriate role in these circumstances?

One option, of course, is to use the Ethical Grid to assist a process of detailed moral reasoning (so overriding the Rings). She might make this move straight away, if she wishes, but it is still possible to discover more precision using only the Rings.

## STEP SIX

The Rings cannot be used abstractly. Dependent upon content and circumstance the importance of any segment will vary. Noting this, further life can be breathed into the Rings by granting movement to the segments, to allow their area to fluctuate in size. The lines dividing the segments can now pivot around the centre-point of the Rings, and can be altered like the hands on a carriage-clock.

Thus it may be that if a nurse manager decides, for a particular case, that there are three key considerations (say technical competence, resources and law) she will not be restricted to a static model of this type (Figure 20).

Instead she will be able to reflect upon her decision by according each consideration a relative importance (Figure 21).

By altering the segments in such a way the manager indicates that her skill and knowledge are the main concern in this case. Her decision about where she stands within the Rings expressed for competence will have a crucial influence on the decision taken.

## Scoring and Quantification

The Rings of Uncertainty are designed primarily as conceptual guidelines, not to provide rigid, quantifiable rulings. However, it might be that individual health workers will wish to invent a personal scoring system, particularly if their specialisation is such that they tend to conceive most or all of their markers placed neither in the centre nor on the outside of the Rings whenever they have to make a decision. It may be that for some a system of numbers could prove decisive in

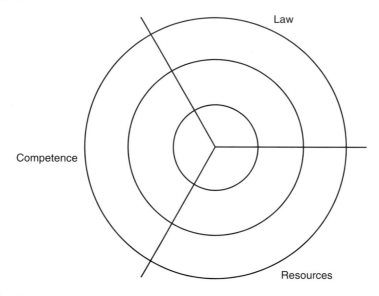

**Figure 20**   Static segments

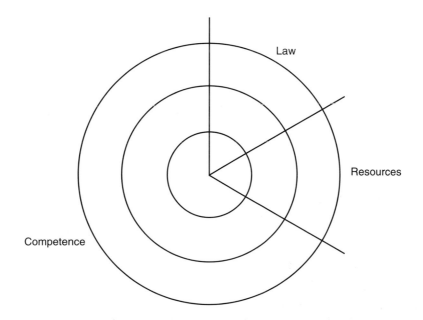

**Figure 21**   Flexible segments

borderline cases, where a doctor (for instance) must choose whether or not to go ahead with an intervention. As one means of orientation a doctor might decide to score the centre of the Rings as four, the next ring as three, the outer ring as two, and the surrounding area as zero. She might decide she will add up the scores for each ring, divide by the number of segments, and accept a cut-off point of say, less than three, as a guide that she should not proceed. If she chooses a lower cut-off point, then she will be choosing to take greater risks, but may find other benefits along the way.

To act as a reasonable guide the Rings must be precise enough to generate some sort of score, but flexible enough to reflect the fact that deliberation about health care frequently transcends crude counting. This system must always take the vagaries of life into account – the aspects of care which cannot be effectively modelled. For instance, dependent upon the context it may not always be a disadvantage for a health worker to be standing in the outer circles for the Rings expressed for competence, ethics and law. So to score less than three, or less than whatever other figure has been selected, need not imply that a halt must be called. In order for a health worker to assess properly whether or not to intervene he must have thought through his priorities, he must be clear about the main theoretical drives of his practice. The primary purpose of the Rings of Uncertainty is not to offer a dubious 'ideal solution' to the question, 'at what point, for how long, and in what way should I intervene?' The Rings are meant to move their users to the point where they recognise it is essential to have a coherent opinion about the importance of their work, and also to offer a logical starting point for the development of such a rationale.

## A Further Educational Use

The scoring system can be used to review the past performances of any health worker, as a learning experience, to enable her to consider whether or not she should have practised as she did. Or if this is too threatening the scoring system could be used to assess hypothetical health workers in invented cases.

# THREE CASE STUDIES TO SHOW THE FULL VALUE OF THE RINGS

---

### 16.   USING THE RINGS OF UNCERTAINTY FULLY EXPRESSED

*Consider this difficult medical situation, and imagine how a doctor might deal with it by employing the Rings as an aid to his deliberation.*

Dr Wilson is a consultant paediatrician facing an unpleasant problem. He is responsible for the care of a severely handicapped neonate – a week-old infant. The baby has an inoperable condition but, with prolonged intensive care stands a 50% chance of surviving, for a few years at least. However, it is likely that his distress – both mental and physical – will be so great that many people would not judge his life to be worth living. The baby's parents – both Catholic – are desperately distressed.

_____ *continues* _____

*continued*

As a general rule Dr Wilson concerns himself only with patients who are actually in his care. He believes he cannot be expected to consider potential patients as well – even though because of lack of facilities he may have to turn away some who have better chances than his current charges. The doctor is accustomed to dramatic medicine, and often makes 'heroic' interventions. He believes 'death with dignity' a crucial concept for his branch of medicine, that 'letting die' is fundamentally different from 'killing', and is preferable by far.

However, Dr Wilson is a thoughtful man, inclined to reassess his position periodically. He decides his present dilemma – which is whether or not to continue intensive care for this baby – provides good opportunity for a re-examination of his motives and role. He resolves to picture himself within the Rings of Uncertainty.

The primary issue here is not 'What should I do?', although this is a question he must answer, but 'What is my proper role here? To what extent ought I intervene in this situation? To what extent am I equipped to undertake the various options?'

## THE RINGS EXPRESSED

Dr Wilson considers that he needs to use all the available segments: competence, resources, law, communication and ethics. Thus he has an initial picture of the Rings as shown in Figure 22.

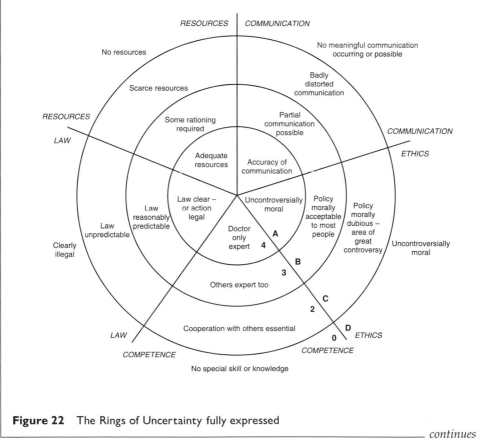

**Figure 22**   The Rings of Uncertainty fully expressed

*continues*

*continued*

Dr Wilson is not sure, before he has thought the problem through, how large each segment should be – so he decides to leave them roughly equal. Even the relative importance of the elements of the problem is uncertain at this stage.

*How can Dr Wilson perceive his position? How is he to determine his proper role in this case? What should limit his practice?*

Clearly there are several considerations, potential limits, and possible courses of action in play. Not all the options will be of the same merit, but he might choose more than one.

Dr Wilson begins to explore the Rings. Logically enough he begins in the competence segment. Now, if Dr Wilson sees himself standing outside the Rings – where he has no special skill or knowledge – he should stop his deliberation at this initial thought. If he is not competent to make the decision he should pass the problem over to someone else, or to a team of people. Perhaps a nurse, a priest, a philosopher or the parents will be better equipped to make the best decision.

In fact Dr Wilson is not so unassuming. He tentatively places himself within the second circle from the centre (B), thus acknowledging that others are expert too. But he is careful not to annul his option to assert his authority, if he thinks it necessary. By picturing himself standing in this part-circle for the Rings expressed for technical competence Dr Wilson has retained the right to continue to reflect about his role. He does not accept that his less-than-perfect competence to make this judgement should limit him. He may not be right, however. He is deliberating only with himself. He may face a tougher test to establish his claim to a role in conversation with others.

He worries about the law. He is profoundly aware of the Arthur case[74] and of Re B.[75] As he understands the law, if he were to kill the baby by poisoning him, then he might run the risk of a charge of murder. If he intends active euthanasia, then the law is a serious restriction. But this is not his intention.

Dr Wilson has long held the belief that to discontinue treatment is not a positive act (although not everyone shares this view).[76] For him not doing something is not morally equivalent to doing something. If there were no medical facilities the baby would not be alive in any case. Not to treat is natural, he thinks. Doctors are not 'Gods'. Sometimes it is better to 'let nature take its course'. Dr Wilson is also familiar with many precedents for this (he has made similar interventions in the past, and he is reassured that Dr Arthur was not found guilty). However, he recognises some risk of legal action and so places himself in the second innermost Ring (B), since he regards the law as only reasonably predictable.

He knows he ought to involve the parents if at all possible, at the very least to ascertain their wishes. However, there are tremendous problems of communication. Both parents regard life as sacred, but both are also acutely aware of the horrifying condition of their baby. They are crying, grieving already, and their competence to reason calmly is obviously diminished. In addition, it is hard for all concerned to discuss ending the life of such a young and vulnerable being. Consequently Dr Wilson decides to close up the communication segment, making it comparatively small – he doesn't regard it as particularly important and places himself in the outer circle of the small segment (C) in the belief that communication will inevitably be badly distorted. Dr Wilson also thinks that since he has considered the possibility that the parents might have as much expertise as he does, and has found them to be temporarily incapacitated, he must now see himself as standing within the centre circle for technical competence (A), moving inwards one circle. Only he is expert at this decision now. He feels that if he decides to discontinue treatment (which is his inclination) then it will be important to ensure that the parents do not suffer guilt – he will prevent this burden at least.

*continues*

*continued*

At this point Dr Wilson would certainly face a strong challenge from other quarters. He does not have privileged access to some 'moral truth', and it is not out of the question that a stronger justification might be advanced for an alternative policy. However, the purpose of describing a doctor reflecting upon his position within the Rings of Uncertainty is to display the working of the process rather than to advance a moral argument.

Dr Wilson's resources are adequate. He is within the centre circle for this segment – he has time, staff, equipment, and finance. Treatment is available for the child, if it is considered appropriate. Afterwards, however, if the baby survives he will continue to need expensive care. Even later there will be a significant demand on state resources to maintain and support the infant.

Dr Wilson looks at the image he has produced and sees he has not only clarified the situation but arrived at a decision. His image looks like this:

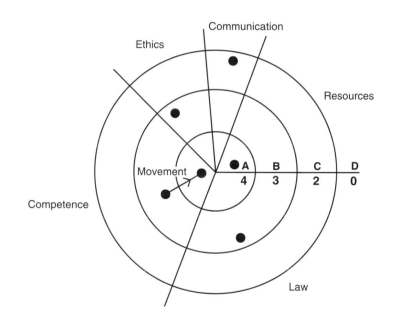

**Figure 23**   Dr Wilson's picture

According to his personal scoring system the doctor feels he should – in the best interest of the child and his parents – discontinue intensive care. He thinks this would be acceptable to most people, especially if they could witness his deformities and suffering. He realises he does not know this for sure, and is aware that whatever decision he takes will be contentious.

He scores 16 divided by 5, an average score of over 3 – so he is reassured he has a role (which was the major part of his initial question). He is operating within a variety of

*continues*

*continued*

uncertainties. In addition to his uncertainties of interpretation, of ethics, and of self, he does not know what will happen to the child if therapy is discontinued. Dr Wilson is clear, however, that he is operating within the limits of medicine. 'Who else', he asks, 'could take such a decision?'

Other people might place Dr Wilson in different circles, and set the segments to different sizes. However, because Dr Wilson has produced a clear, graphic image, because he has made his deliberation about the extent of his role overt and explicit, the use of the Rings at least allows meaningful conversation to start.

The case of the badly handicapped neonate is not one which can have a happy solution. Whatever the decision, there will be tragedy. A more complete ethical analysis would involve a detailed consideration of the range of cost and benefits, a discussion of the doctor's duty and priorities, and an assessment of the severity of the various potential harms (or dwarfings) with a view to minimising them. In other words, a full analysis requires the Ethical Grid.

## EXERCISE

1. Do you agree with Dr Wilson's decision and use of the Rings?

2. Return to this question once you can use the Ethical Grid competently. Use the Grid to help you deliberate as if you are Dr Wilson.

3. Do you now agree with Dr Wilson's decision and use of the Rings?

## 17.   LIVE OR LET DIE? – UNCERTAINTY OF ROLE

Consider an emotionally fraught disagreement between two adult children about the treatment of their dying mother.

The mother is in her eighties. Two years ago she suffered a severe stroke which paralysed one side of her body. Between then and now she has been cared for full-time by her 48-year-old daughter. The son has a home in America, where he works as an engineer.

The mother has contracted pneumonia, and is semi-comatose. On diagnosing the condition the doctor speaks to both son and daughter, outlining the options, which are: do nothing (in which case death is likely in days); treat with antibiotics at home (in which case the infection may clear, though it will probably return shortly); to treat 'aggressively' in hospital (in which case the infection may be resisted for longer). The daughter, feeling that her mother is no longer 'properly alive', wants no intervention. However the son wants 'everything possible' done to save his mother.
The doctor counsels both offspring, who fail to reach agreement. The doctor then calls in key relatives, including the sister of the sick woman, who eventually persuade the son to concur with his sister.

*continues*

continued

Setting aside discussion about the morality of euthanasia, the central issue in this case is the role of the doctor. At present her clinical training equips her to diagnose the condition, and prescribe appropriate treatment. It does not, usually, equip her to counsel. It certainly does not legitimise interventions beyond the treatment of disease, and certainly not into the lives of others who have no disease. It is fair to say, 'What else could she do in such a situation?' But it is nonetheless important to recognise the need for clarification of the doctor's role.

## EXERCISE

Consider the limits of the doctor's role by the use of the Rings of Uncertainty fully expressed. Include any further background details you feel necessary – or imagine yourself to be the doctor in question tackling a similar case.

Having thus clarified the situation analyse it with the benefit of the Ethical Grid, once you have it mastered. What should the doctor have done to create the highest degree of morality?

## 18.   DEALING WITH DYING

If this exercise is to be used for either a role or thought play then select a character.

## The Characters

Louise (a woman close to death from cancer)

Daniel (her son)

Dr Jonathan Cook (senior lecturer in oncology – cancer specialist)

Marianne (an SRN on Ward Twelve)

### Louise

Louise is a widow of 48 first diagnosed with breast cancer four years ago. She underwent a radical mastectomy followed by radiotherapy and chemotherapy. Two years later a recurrence was found in her lymph node. Now a brain secondary has been confirmed. Louise has been admitted to Ward Twelve, often used to house terminally ill patients, although other people with cancers are also cared for here. Louise has been a patient on this ward three times before.

Louise has not been told explicitly by anyone that she has a brain secondary. However she feels prepared for death, but has not yet been able to talk about her mortality with anyone in her family other than her sister, with whom she has often stayed during her illness years. She told Dr Cook a few months ago he was not to continue treating her just to keep her alive when things became hopeless.

continues

continued

It is almost Christmas, and the ward is plastered with tinsel, greeting cards and plastic images of Santa Claus. Christmas has a reassuring continuity which Louise thinks is nice. She feels surrounded by other Christmases. Images of her late husband, and a house full of excited children expecting carloads of friends and relatives, pass through her mind.

Louise feels in a daze. She is often confused, and fully lucid only intermittently. When she can make sense she seems to talk more as a little girl than a woman. But this is some sort of defence, helped by her painkilling drugs. She knows she is dying, and feels indescribably tired, though when she becomes more alert she seems to come back to life. Then she expresses regret at her passivity, she 'doesn't know what came over her', and reasserts her determination to fight, to get better soon. Louise is a chaos of emotions, a cocktail of denial, resistance and acceptance.

When she accepts she can think only of a single wish, which she has not the strength to fulfil. She simply wishes she could tell Daniel she loves him.

## Daniel

Daniel is 24, the eldest of Louise's three children. By coincidence he lives close to the hospital where his mother is being treated, while his brother and sister live over 90 miles away. He feels he must somehow assume responsibility as the chief next-of-kin of his mother, and so he visits her every day.

Daniel feels he is a disappointment to his mother. As a youth he was far more interested in having a good time than in study or a career. But he is now in his second year at the local university where he is a mature student. It took a lot of work and self-control to get there and he wishes his mother would acknowledge his recent efforts. He believes (with justification) his mother sees him as 'the bad sheep' – a bit of a waster.

Daniel feels numb. He knows his Mum must die soon, but cannot grasp this as a reality. He cannot picture his mother dying. Looking out of the window of the bus to the hospital each day the world seems more distant than it used to be, as if he were an observer not really taking part in any of it. During his visits the conversation is slow and sparse. Mother and son talk about plants and pets, which are mutual interests, but nothing more important. He feels he would like to express everything he has ever felt for his mother: his anger, his frustration, his need for approval, his sorrow for hurting her, but he cannot even get so far as to think 'I need to tell her I love her'. When he is with her he closes in on himself.

## Dr Jonathan Cook

Dr Cook is a senior doctor. He has vast experience of cancer treatment and prognosis, and of the medical care of the dying. He is a hard-working academic and a kind man. Dr Cook thinks Louise is an exceptional patient. He believes that without her determination she would have been dead two years ago, but she is a fighter and he knows how important that is in cancer patients.

Dr Cook is also fond of Louise. He is a similar age, and from a similar background. They have had some frank conversations during the treatment programme, but now he feels less able to be open.

He has not thought through the reasons why his attitude has changed, but has withdrawn rapidly from the relationship with the dying woman. He now keeps a 'professional distance' and leaves virtually all the care to the nursing staff. He has, and still has every day, the opportunity to tell her that she definitely has a brain tumour, and

continues

_ continued _

is approaching death. But he doesn't do it. Louise is now under the direct care of a more junior doctor. Dr Cook feels that speaking to Louise is no longer his role. If the other doctor wishes to tell her then that is for him to decide.

## Marianne

Marianne hates this ward. She finds it desperately stressful to have to nurse people who are dying and often in great distress. She has applied for a transfer to intensive care where there is at least as much stress, but where people do sometimes recover. Marianne has been nursing Louise for three weeks, and is truly torn by the experience. When Louise is lucid and talking of getting better and going home, Marianne feels very close to her. Louise has a sweet nature which reminds Marianne of her own mother. But when Louise is in decline, Marianne just wishes she wouldn't wake up.

Marianne has observed the relationship between Louise and her son, and is familiar with their communication difficulties. She can see they are exceptionally bad at it, and it upsets her.

Marianne is always cheerful on the surface, always the jolly nurse. Daniel scowls at her when he sees her. He thinks her gaiety is quite inappropriate, just like the elaborate Christmas decor. Marianne doesn't know this. She thinks he is an unpleasant and inadequate young man. Why doesn't he just hold his mother's hand for Chrissake?

Marianne has spoken to the social worker to ask her to speak to Daniel. She doesn't feel able to speak to Daniel and Louise herself, though she would dearly like to try to encourage them to talk to resolve their relationship.

## The Situation

There is a crisis. Daniel has come for an afternoon visit. Louise is drowsy, but conscious. She is lying on her side, breathing wheezily. She seems very warm to Daniel as he leans over her to whisper hello. He is surprised to notice she seems to smell of babies. As he moves to find a chair he spots that her saline drip has gone. He is pleased, he feels a surge of hope. But then he thinks again, as he sits quiet and still. A middle-aged woman in the bed opposite catches his eye, and starts to talk to him.

'It's a shame, it's a shame, it really is. She's not very old...neither are you. It's a shame. I know her well you know. We were in here together last year. Oh...it really is a shame...'

What's she talking like this for? Daniel jumps up in instant fear. He runs to the desk. He asks Marianne what's happening (he doesn't know her name). She says she isn't sure (though she is). Dr Cook has said Louise is not to be disturbed any more. She's not to have any more medication.

'Where is he? I want to see him. Please.' Daniel is first polite, then begins to shout. 'Where is that bloody doctor? I want him here now. He doesn't know what he is doing. Come on. I'm not leaving until he comes. Please get him here. Get him here.' Becoming increasingly agitated, Daniel leans over the desk and begins to push notes and files to the floor.

*EXERCISE*

1. Imagine the situation up to now from the point of view of your selected character. Try hard to imagine the situation from the points of view of other characters.

2. Now act out in your imagination what happens next, playing the part of your selected character. Imagine the situation from the points of view of other characters.

3. If in a class with others, act out the situation as a role play.

What are the main implications of this situation? What should the roles of the doctor and nurse be? What skills might they need?

## USING THE RINGS FULLY EXPRESSED

1. Select a character (either Dr Cook or Marianne).

2. Decide what to do next.

3. Using the Rings fully expressed (see Figure 22) place markers/picture yourself within the Rings. If you like, calculate the level of risk of your plan. Remember you can alter the size of the segments.

Examples: Marianne might decide to expel Daniel from the ward. She may attempt to do this herself.

Dr Cook might agree to recommence treatment.

Dr Cook and Marianne might decide to call on others – perhaps including Social Work staff – for help.

## USING THE ETHICAL GRID

Imagine you are Marianne. Devise a strategy to create the highest degree of morality. Criticise your scheme as rigorously as you can, using as much of the Grid as possible.

# CHAPTER TEN

# The Background to the Ethical Grid

## AN ANALOGY

The Ethical Grid is not a conveyer belt. It does not deliver correct answers in neat packages – rather it is like a gardener's spade. Like a good gardener, the proficient Grid user understands the importance of keeping her tool clean and sharp. Whether the implement is a spade or the Grid, and whether it is employed on soil or persons, the good worker will recognise when to use it. Sometimes conditions are unsuitable – the ground may be waterlogged, or the law or a social policy clear and agreed (though even in these cases it is worth trying the Grid out, to see what it reveals). Furthermore, the end results of even the most masterful use of either tool are never entirely predictable. Even with the most conscientious practice there is no guarantee that a particular digging method (and there is a range of options open to gardeners) will produce the desired horticultural results, and it is equally possible that even the most painstaking use of the Grid may not spawn the best practical results.

## WHAT IS THE GRID AND HOW DOES IT WORK?

On referring to the figure of the complete Grid (Figure 30, on p. 209) the following features will be noticed:

1. There are four different layers to the Grid, indicated by different colours (blue, red, green, and black).
2. Each of the boxes, whatever its colour, is self-contained and detachable.
3. The Grid can be seen in more than one way. It is possible to use it as if the coloured layers have to be addressed in a set order. For instance, a user might think the most significant principles are those contained in the blue boxes at the centre of the Grid, and that the outer boxes are of decreasing importance as one steps (or spirals if that is the preferred method) to the outer limit of the Grid. But this use is not necessarily always the most appropriate.

   Alternatively a user might follow a spiral running from the outer limit of the Grid into the blue core, or might always begin with a consideration of consequences, or might always consider – as a start – four specific boxes, one taken from each coloured layer.

The Grid can also be seen as either a two- or three-dimensional object. If it is envisaged in three dimensions the four sides of the pyramid might be considered in turn. However, there is no special relationship or association between the boxes on each side.

Even if the Grid is seen in two dimensions it need not remain static on the page. It can be flexible in the user's imagination. For instance, it is possible to imagine an invisible cord at its centre which can pull the Grid (as if written on a piece of rubber) either towards or away from the viewer. The direction of the pull will depend upon the importance a user wishes to accord to the various layers. In this way the Grid can remain in view and in mind as a whole, though it should be noted that this use has less pliancy than regarding each box as detachable.

4. The Grid has to be applied to practical cases for it to come to life.


## WHY IS THE GRID COMPOSED OF DIFFERENT COLOURED LAYERS?

First of all it must be explained that the Grid is an artificial device, and the separation of boxes into apparently airtight compartments is also artificial. Nor is it suggested that the Ethical Grid is an exact representation of the mental processes that make up moral reasoning, which is by no means as precise a process as the Grid might make it appear. However, in order to provide health workers with a practical and accessible route into moral reasoning, the layers have been distinguished by the use of colour. Given time and experience it ought not be necessary to refer to the Grid at all – it is certainly not a substitute for moral reasoning. Yet even the most seasoned moral thinker might find it useful to refer back to the Grid from time to time, to remind herself of the elements that should be part of a thorough deliberation.

The Grid is presented in four layers to show that at least four aspects are necessary to comprehensive ethical analysis. A deliberation which examines only the consequences of actions, or only the law, or only duties might happen to produce good results, but it will not have been carried through with integrity. Furthermore, *health work deliberations should, if the resulting actions are to be health work at all, refer to at least one box from the blue layer*.

It is not suggested that before every intervention the health worker pulls out his 'pocket Ethical Grid' and selects boxes until he is satisfied he has the right combination. This would be quite impractical. Nor is it claimed that the Grid is an indispensable advance in ethical reasoning. But it does make some of the processes of moral reasoning clearer for those unfamiliar with this way of thinking, and as such it is an aid both to understanding and to confidence. The thoughtful health worker can first become familiar with the Grid and its use by practising on hypothetical cases, and then by applying it to cases in practice where there is sufficient time. Proficiency in moral reasoning will improve with practice.

The Ethical Grid has been constructed with health professionals in mind, but it could also be used by people who are not paid to work for health. Work for health in its richest sense is work every member of a society can be involved in.

# THE BLUE LAYER

The blue layer (Figure 26, on p. 204) is set at the centre of the Grid because it is its core rationale. Its four boxes represent – in the most basic manner – the key components of the foundations theory of health.[1,5] The Ethical Grid should be seen as a practical manifestation of this theory.

## CREATE AUTONOMY

### What is Autonomy? (brief answer)

Why is the creation of autonomy a central part of work for health? This question may be answered quickly in two complementary ways: by focusing on practical tradition, and by studying other theories of health.

#### The Historical Tradition

Whatever the means, whether through a personal regime of living or a medical and health professional intervention, practical work for health has always been carried out with the intention of creating autonomy. If treatments are not designed with this end in mind there is little point in making them at all.

A broken arm is a physical impediment to autonomy, and also an obstacle to biological development. Unless it is excruciatingly painful a broken arm does not undermine autonomy completely – a wide range of choices and possibilities will often remain – but it does restrict personal possibility to a degree. An intervention to mend a broken arm is obviously carried out in order to remove the obstacle to normal biological development, but this is not the only reason; it is also carried out in order to enable the person to move on in life without the obstacle. In other words the health intervention is done in order to allow a person the maximum degree of autonomy. The whole point of humane treatment is to enable full persons to flourish as much as possible.

The principle of autonomy has, as a matter of fact, always inspired health work.

#### All Plausible Theories of Health Equate Work for Health, in Some Way, with the Creation of Autonomy

In a previous work[1] a variety of theories of health are presented and discussed. Among the most influential are: the theory that health is an ideal state, the theory that a person is healthy if she can function in a socially useful role, the theory that health can be bought or given as if it is a commodity, and the theory that health is an ability or strength to adapt to the changing challenges and circumstances of life. Though these theories do not share a common view of health, each makes good sense up to a point – and each incorporates the idea of autonomy to some degree. For instance, the World Health Organisation's 'ideal state' is one in which a person is physically, mentally, and socially well, has a satisfying life, and can be economically productive – all notions which require a good level of autonomy. Autonomy is obviously required to carry out a socially useful role (although the level needed will vary dependent upon the role and the society), and the giving or selling of medical commodities – though done for a variety of reasons – is nevertheless valuable in direct proportion to the increased autonomy brought about in the receivers or purchasers of the commodities. Finally, the ability to adapt to life's changing circumstances is actually a general definition of autonomy, according to which health just is personal autonomy, and work for health the creation of an ability to thrive (or at least persevere) whatever trauma is suffered.

(Note: readers who wish to learn the content of the other three blue boxes and the remaining layers of the Ethical Grid directly, should turn to p. 202. But for a detailed, practical account of the importance of autonomy, read on.)

## What is Autonomy? (detailed answer)

Several ethical principles have been hailed as health care's primary inspiration. 'Being just', 'not doing harm', and 'doing positive good' are all candidates.[77] At times each can assume temporary precedence over competing notions, even when some forms of autonomy are at stake. For example, when a resource is scarce not all 'autonomy claims' can be met and just distribution must be the priority. Nevertheless, autonomy is the pivotal health care notion.

## Autonomy is Basic to Health Care

To say autonomy has no importance in health care is a contradiction in terms:

1. Under Western law consent is essential in any health care intervention which involves touching a competent person. Without consent, touching is a civil or criminal offence. In order for a person to consent to an operation he must have sufficient knowledge to understand the implications of what is proposed. To put it another way, his level of autonomy must be sufficient to give him command of the decision.
2. There is no difference in kind between the problem of disease and other problems of life – there is difference of degree only. All problems affect an individual's autonomy – when a person has a problem her autonomy is lessened by definition, at least in the part of her life where the problem exists. Because disease is not radically different from other problems, health workers have no special obligation or right to fight it. Any justification of work against disease must refer to the creation of autonomy, since this is fundamental.
3. Work for health is work to liberate enhancing human potentials. This enhancement is necessarily the creation of autonomy. Health work can diminish only when this diminishing avoids worse harms.
4. Unless an arbitrary distinction is made between physical and mental mobility, if autonomy is a priority then physical and mental autonomy matter equally.

These four points make most sense once a distinction between different understandings of autonomy is grasped. There is Understanding A – *autonomy as being able to do* – and Understanding B – *autonomy as being able to have one's expressed wants*. These categories are explained during the course of this section.

Autonomy is not health work's only inspiration. In complicated situations extensive deliberation is required (the Ethical Grid is meant to support precisely this). However, interventions which make no attempt to increase autonomy are not health work.[78]

# THE RICHNESS OF AUTONOMY

In most medical ethics literature an 'autonomous person' is said to be 'self-determining' – to have control of her destiny. Autonomy is taken to involve personal wants – an autonomous person can determine what she desires and if her autonomy is respected no one will stand in her way. But this is Understanding B only. It fails to grasp the depth of autonomy's meaning.

There are at least three different ways of thinking about autonomy.

## AUTONOMY AS A SINGLE PRINCIPLE

On this understanding autonomy is a principle that 'the wishes of individuals ought to be respected'. Critics of the use of this principle[79] point out that 'autonomy is not the only ethical imperative'. Such commentators are quite correct to say that in some circumstances other considerations take precedence over the desires of individuals (for instance, if a person has irrational desires, or if his desires will cause avoidable harm to others) but wrong to believe they have therefore exposed the limitations of the concept. They have not, because autonomy should be thought of more broadly.

The mistaken devaluation of autonomy is common within the pages of some medical journals, particularly in papers on 'ethics in medicine' by doctors who lack philosophical education. For example, a paper in the *Journal of the Royal College of General Practitioners*[80] asked doctors to say what they would do in brief vignettes about control of information in 'unhealthy lifestyle'. The authors chose to offer 'patient welfare' and 'patient autonomy' as contrasting reasons for action. But by separating welfare and autonomy like this the authors assume 'autonomy' means nothing more than 'patient control of decision-making'. If so the only question is: does the principle of autonomy apply in this case, or is it better that the doctor decides? Not only is this a very crude representation of clinical reality (where education, conversation, coercion, guilt and recrimination often subtly combine) but it reflects little of autonomy's real meaning. In fact, as we shall see, concern for patient welfare is itself a central part of autonomy creation.

## AUTONOMY AS A RIGHT

The view that autonomy is a principle has led many writers to claim that autonomy is a right. To assert the right to autonomy is to declare that people capable of self-determination ought not be manipulated, even if others believe this is in their best interest. This is a plausible view of autonomy, but again it is too simple. It regards autonomy as a single type of thing (like life or property – which you either have or have not) which everyone – apart from those whose thought processes are disabled for one reason or another – should have.

This makes perfect fighting sense where people are repressed, where human beings are not allowed self-determination and creative self-expression, and where they might be freed. In such cases to speak of the right to autonomy can be a powerful and emotive weapon. In these circumstances one might justly scream – these people have a right to autonomy! But although this may be politically effective it is impossible to demonstrate that moral rights exist. We have many legal rights, but laws are invented. No one can show conclusively that 'human rights' exist in any form other than human convention. We do not have an objective right to life, we merely have life. Despite volumes of writing on the subject,[81] to cast argument for change in rights language is philosophically unhelpful. To speak of autonomy as a right is to do nothing more than to say 'I believe that the human ability to choose should be acknowledged and personal choices respected'. However often this is said, and by however many people, autonomy does not move one jot nearer to becoming an objective right. To speak of autonomy as if it is a right is to perpetuate the myth that autonomy is a single state and something that can be attained or ceded.

## AUTONOMY AS A QUALITY

Autonomy is essentially a quality, not a disembodied principle or a right partially separate from human beings. It is utterly wrong to think of autonomy as something that is entirely lost if a right to choose is denied.

Rather autonomy is an intrinsic personal quality. At its most basic, *to be autonomous is to be able to do – to be able to do anything rather than nothing*. Autonomy, thought of in this way, is a matter of degree – the better the quality of the autonomy the more a person is able to do. A person becomes able to move more extensively in her life as her level of autonomy rises.

This view of autonomy is more complicated than the other versions, and requires detailed explanation. The remainder of this chapter is devoted to this task. By thinking of autonomy as a quality it is possible to move forward on several fronts. It becomes possible to:

1. Make a clear distinction between *creating autonomy* and *respecting autonomy*.
2. Show conclusively that respecting autonomy in the sense of 'agreeing to the wishes of others' (a derivative of Understanding B) is a weak idea without reference to the creation or increase of autonomy (Understanding A). When autonomy is conceived of as a basic quality essential to human dignity, which can be enhanced or diminished dependent upon what happens to or is done to people, then work to increase autonomy becomes work to raise the level of human possibility. More prosaically, in a medical context it may be that a doctor considers he is abiding by the principle of autonomy and respecting a patient's right to autonomy in full so long as he is neutral and does not place undue influence upon him. It is not uncommon to hear doctors argue that a *laissez-faire* approach shows sufficient regard for autonomy – 'the main thing is to let the patient make up her own mind'

and 'it's not always up to me to tell the patient everything about his condition – if he wants to know he will ask'. But without additional help this may not be enough – the patient may not have a high enough level of autonomy. Her autonomy may not yet be of a quality good enough to enable her to exercise a reasoned choice.

Indeed, if doctors think respecting autonomy merely means saying 'over to you' whenever there are hard clinical decisions to be taken, they have things badly wrong. Superficially it may seem as if a patient's 'right' to exercise the 'principle' is respected if she is left alone to decide to have treatment or not. Certainly she will not be under pressure to do what clinicians would like, but without advice, support and education – and especially if she is upset and anxious – she may have little or no autonomy to exercise.

3. List ways of enhancing autonomy and contrast these to diminishings or constrainings. In this regard it is important to recognise that the quality of autonomy can be improved or worsened by factors internal to a person – factors at least partly within the power of individuals – and also by external factors.
4. Demonstrate that in health work there is a crucial point at which efforts to create autonomy (Understanding A) – efforts to improve the quality of a person's autonomy by trying to enhance what that person is able to do – become secondary to a duty to respect autonomy in the sense urged by talk of principles and rights (Understanding B). It can be shown that an *autonomy flip* can occur, where work to create autonomy must give way to respect for autonomy.
5. Begin to consider solutions to a seemingly intractable dilemma. This occurs whenever it is felt more important to provide for a person's welfare (creating autonomy in line with Understanding A) than to respond to a person's expressed wants (respecting autonomy in line with Understanding B). One trivial example of this dilemma occurs when a decision is made to deny fat children sticky buns even though they want them. A perhaps more serious example confronts doctors who work with people who experience problems with illicit drug use. Should doctors provide the drugs cheaply and safely – which is what many drug users want – or should they insist on detoxification out of concern for their welfare? Which policy has most regard for autonomy?

(Note: It is true to say that if it is argued that autonomy is a quality, and that this quality ought to be increased, then this belief could be translated into a principle. Equally, if health workers have a duty to enhance this quality in others, then it might be argued that this implies a right to have one's autonomy increased.

The first suggestion is undoubtedly true – we create principles and there is no reason why we should not create this one. However, we must remember that the principle is not a thing in itself but originates from admiration of a complex human quality.

The second recommendation is a little more complicated. If it is meant to imply an objective right, then it is wrong. The duty to create autonomy stems from health workers' decisions to commit to work for health, and does not exist before this pledge. Furthermore, a health worker does not have an indefinite duty to create autonomy, but is limited by her understanding of health. No one has an absolute right to have her autonomy increased.)

# AUTONOMY AS A HUMAN QUALITY

The view that autonomy is a human quality stems from the foundations theory of health,[1,5] according to which work for health is supposed to remove obstacles in the way of human potential. Not all of these can be eliminated by cutting away. Some can be removed only through the provision of something else. For instance, ignorance is an obstacle that can be remedied only by giving information. Work for health, thought of in this sense, is work to enable, work to provide a stage on which to perform. The greater a person's stage the more movement in life she will have.

This view of health must explain autonomy as a quality. Because health is directly related to the freedom of body and mind, and not necessarily associated with freedom from disease and illness, autonomy does not just mean the ability of a person to command her physicians. According to the foundations theory of health autonomy makes full sense only when it means being able to do in the widest sense.

There are degrees of autonomy as a quality – it is not something one either has or has not – and it is a complex notion. A person may be highly autonomous in some respects and incompetent in others. Autonomy is not, however, necessarily related to the amount of options available. Much depends upon context. A physically disabled child living in poverty with an uncaring family – a child living in conditions which disadvantage him on top of his handicap – will have a lower level of autonomy than a physically fit, loved, exceptionally talented Eton schoolboy. However it does not always follow that wealth, age, or fitness are connected to levels of autonomy. For example, a 5-year-old child will not have the same range of options as a 30-year-old middle-class insurance executive – he will not usually be able to do as much as freely – but the child will still be able to exert some control in the aspects of his life which matter most to him. For instance, he will probably be able to choose which toys he plays with, and which books he reads – within a range of options. Realistically, taking account of the different contexts of the two people, their levels of autonomy – the quality of what they might do – can be said to be roughly equivalent.

Whoever we are, whatever circumstances we live under, we are all (unless permanently comatose) able to do some things – able to move freely in some areas of life – and constrained in other aspects. These constraints can be internal to us (for example, limit of talent, limit of willpower) or external (for example, restrictions created by the desires of others, or no resources to allow us to travel widely).

Thus it makes good sense to see autonomy as the ability to do, a quality almost all of us possess to some degree, and a quality which can frequently be enhanced in a great range of ways. This insight shows it is possible to work to increase autonomy without having to be a docile pawn in the game of another person. It is possible to work for autonomy in this broad sense without always having to do what another person requests. And this turns out to be a very important distinction.

Creating autonomy – enhancing the human quality of doing – is basic to health care. It is possible to represent the basic ground of work for autonomy in this way. Autonomy increases as a person moves towards the right of the spectrum.

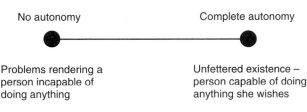

**Figure 24**  The basic autonomy spectrum

Work to create autonomy does not necessarily imply obedience to patient choice. It is true to say that the creation of choice is a primary goal, but in many cases work can be undertaken to create autonomy without direct reference to it. For example, it may be that a nurse believes a person's depression might be alleviated by a change in his social life. To a withdrawn and lethargic person such a change might not seem at all desirable. However, if the nurse feels change in the person's social life is genuinely worth trying (and the nurse would need to be able to point to evidence to support her proposal) then, in order to create autonomy, she would be justified in a range of attempts to involve the patient in group activity. Although the nurse would not be respecting personal choice immediately, her intent would be to enable the patient to do more, to be freer from the grip of his depression. Hand in hand with the achievement of this goal the patient would gain a higher level of choice. This is not to say that a health worker can force a person to do something against her expressed wishes, but if there is ambivalence then she may seek to create autonomy – but only with the specific aim of moving the person to a position where she is able to exercise a more fully reasoned choice (a choice free from depression in this case). The judgement about the point at which respecting autonomy (Understanding B) must take precedence over creating autonomy (Understanding A) is neither easy nor precisely measurable. Inevitably there will be a grey area in which there will be controversy about whether or not the autonomy flip (see p. 192) has occurred. It is unlikely any foolproof method exists to assist in this judgement, though the Autonomy Test outlined later in this section can provide some practical help.

In some cases, in cases where a person is severely mentally handicapped, or where a patient is suffering from a mentally disabling illness, the notion of respect for autonomy may have no part to play. However, this does not mean that the issue of autonomy disappears (as the standard medical ethics account has it). On the contrary, autonomy remains as important as ever. Such a degree of handicap means that a person's life will be subject to some very severe constraints – that the person's autonomy will be of poor quality. But if anything in these cases there is all the more reason to seek avenues which enable the person, even within the severe restrictions of circumstance which surround him. When there is very little of a good thing even the smallest addition can be precious.

In many cases there is a clear relationship between the creation of and respect for autonomy. For instance, it is not possible for a person to express a free wish unless she knows what her situation is, unless she knows the possibilities open to her. So if there are three types of surgery available, and the patient thinks there is only one, she may opt for it, but she will have done so with a lower level of autonomy than she might have had. In this way creating autonomy (as enabling mental doing) can be a prerequisite for respecting autonomy (conforming with informed requests).

The fact that wishing depends upon the achievement of a certain level of being able to do – on the provision of certain conditions both for life movement and choice – is even clearer in some other cases. For example, take the case of a frightened, anxious person entering hospital to discuss a future operation. It is possible to be in such a state of nervousness that one cannot think straight. The person may not even be able to comprehend realistically what is being said to him, never mind formulate a coherent view about what to do about his clinical problem. He may, after meeting the consultant in charge, agree to a particular procedure, but since he has not been able to think properly it makes very little sense to say this is what he wants. In order to have any autonomy (on Understanding B) to respect, autonomy (as being able to do – Understanding A) must be raised to a sufficient level. Looked at with reference to the continuum illustrated in Figure 24, the primary task of the health worker is to ensure that the anxious patient moves from A to B on the spectrum (Figure 25).

As a general guide, the impetus of all health care interventions should be first to try to move a person as far to the right of the spectrum as possible, and secondly to move a person past point B on the spectrum at the earliest possible opportunity. Although the exact position of point B is bound to be the subject of some controversy, and must be decided with reference to the particular facts of the case, this does not invalidate the guiding idea.

It must be said that not all health professionals think of their work like this. Those who do not are not working for health on the foundations theory. It is, to be sure, easier and often more efficient not to work as the first priority to move a person from A to B. For one thing the attempt is likely to be time-consuming. But if autonomy is seriously considered an essential goal of work for health, the effort must be made.

## TWO CASES

Consider the following two cases. Both involve consent, although in subtly different ways. Consent might be defined as an expressed agreement to a procedure based on a level of information which would be sufficient to satisfy the giver of that information if he were to be on the receiving end. Bear in mind that consent must be based ultimately in autonomy as ability to do. That is, a person must already be at a certain point – past point B – on the autonomy spectrum to be able to give a consent.

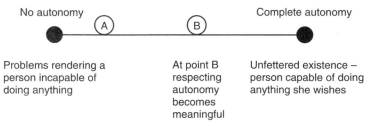

**Figure 25**   The autonomy spectrum indicating a point of 'autonomy flip'

# 19.  CAROLE

Think about Carole, an unemployed, unhappy young woman. She is living in an apparently close middle-class family, which has profound tensions below the surface. Her father is terminally ill.

Carole's behaviour consists of intermittent lethargy, drunkenness and rebellion – but overall she is catastrophically miserable. She gets in trouble with the law, caught shop-lifting a skirt from Marks & Spencer. Carole's parents decide enough is enough, and she is persuaded to see a psychiatrist, who makes a diagnosis but does not tell Carole or her parents what it is. All he will say is that she has an emotional problem she can be helped with. After a couple of weeks in hospital as a 'voluntary patient' Carole is treated as an outpatient. She is given an injection of a long lasting anti-psychotic drug (Modecate) and also another drug (Kemadrin – procyclidine) to counteract possible 'Parkinsonian side-effects'. She is not told what to expect by either the doctor or the nurse who administers the injection.

There are two key issues to consider in this case. *Does Carole give meaningful consent to her treatment, and in which direction is she moved along the autonomy spectrum?* These questions are crucial in the great majority of health care interventions. Before considering answers in Carole's case consider a little more detail. She is having many difficulties in her life, and clearly at a low ebb. Carole is immensely vulnerable. She is blamed by her family and some of her friends for causing most of her troubles – 'Everybody has problems, why does it always have to be you who over-reacts and makes things even worse?' For her own part she blames herself entirely for her calamity.

Carole desperately wants to be happier, to resolve this situation in which she is drowning. She is an intelligent young woman but drifted away from school before taking her final exams – for which she had not worked anyway. Carole has not studied or read anything other than the tabloid newspapers for the last three years: she can't be bothered to read anything else, she can't concentrate and can't see the relevance of any of it to her.

Carole becomes a 'voluntary patient' because she sees it as a way out. She has to do something to get out of the hole and she doesn't have many options left. In addition the pressure placed on her by her family is becoming ever more unbearable. She says she agrees to the drug treatment but she has very little idea what it will do to her, indeed whether it will benefit her in any way (although she knows the demonstration of compliance with her family's wishes might).

The point of this example is not to criticise psychiatry (although something very close to this situation actually happened, culminating in a bemused young person breaking out of a mental hospital through a kitchen window – to escape only to pass out and wake up in the early hours covered in frost) but to show how lack of a theory of health can diminish autonomy. There were clearly many other ways in which Carole's life might have been enhanced, even if the diagnosis had been correct. When disease, or at least perceived disease, is regarded as the priority, above other problems which might receive attention, then it is inevitable that other ways of improving a person's life will neither be spotted nor pursued.

## 20.   EVELYN

The next example is again taken directly from life. It is discussed towards the end of this chapter and presented now as an exercise for self- or group-learning.

### RESEARCH FOR HEALTH?

This case is based on the experience of Evelyn Thomas. Her words have been extracted from an article which appeared in the *Observer* (UK). The reports of the feeling and motivation of the chief researcher are imaginary. The justification offered by the actual researcher can be found elsewhere.[82]

This exercise describes the feelings of two characters. The situation is that a woman who has had a mastectomy has discovered that she has been involved in clinical trials without her consent. The *first trial*, which took place simultaneously in different centres around Britain, involved the testing of preventive hormonal treatment. Evelyn's treatment was compared with that of other women cancer sufferers who were receiving either no further treatment or different drugs.

The *second trial* was to test the effects of post-operative counselling. Evelyn was not counselled yet other patients were. Their 'psychological adjustment' was compared.

We might call the doctor Alan Hughes since the position for which he argues is not unique to the researcher in question. The view advanced below is a paraphrased amalgam of the beliefs of several doctors. It is not intended to represent accurately the opinion of the Professor in real life.

DR HUGHES explains:

'I have been a clinical researcher and consultant surgeon for over 20 years now, and been in medicine for 10 years before that. My experience allows me to balance, in the broadest perspective, long-term human gain against possible short-term individual suffering. I would emphasise my choice of the word "possible". The whole point of research is that the answer is not known. It may turn out that the subject of a controlled trial might have benefited more from a treatment from which she was excluded, but equally she might not have done. We simply do not know for sure, which is why we need to experiment.

'I know that this patient, and you could say the same of others in the past, feels hurt and perhaps abused by what I have done, but I stand by my actions and refuse to change my practice. If this patient had been informed that she was in either trial it would have rendered her inclusion scientifically invalid. We do not know the precise relationship between mental state and physical well-being, and this might have affected our results. This is particularly obvious in the case of the post-operative counselling. We were searching for very specific information, and only this information. This made it necessary for us to control as many variables as possible.

'I think there are three main points to consider here: first of all each research proposal has to be passed – approved – by an ethics committee. These are committees made up of highly experienced, eminent, honourable people. Ethics committees make sure that no research proposal which is at all unethical is passed. They did not consider that I needed consent for my research because they weighed up the costs and benefits, and appreciated the considerable amount of good that potentially could be achieved by the work.

'This raises the second point: if clinical research is permitted only if patients are informed, then we would not have the benefit of many scientific advances. It is vital that we advance our scientific understanding for the benefit of all future patients, and any one of us might be future patients. It must also be said that most people included in research trials do not suffer. In this case no worse treatment was given to the patient. We believed that both drug treatments were roughly equivalent.

_____ *continues* ___|

*continued*

'As for the counselling trial, the patient received the highest standard of care possible from our doctors and nursing staff. It is true to say that she did not receive this particular form of intervention – but at the time we had no idea whether she would benefit from it or find it to her disadvantage. In any case different people respond in different ways to all forms of medical treatment: medicine is the most uncertain of all sciences – there are always exceptions to all forms of treatment, always people who recover when they seem to have no chance of doing so.

'It is also very pertinent to consider what it means to be working at this level in medicine. I cannot just sit still and rest on my laurels. I have to achieve, I have to compete. Some of my younger colleagues – men still in their forties – have published over 300 scientific papers and I have just over 150. I am ambitious and it is expected of me – it is an integral part of the profession that I am involved in. It is unrealistic to expect me to stop doing what so many of my peers are doing: it is part of the profession. Why should I challenge this practice, especially since I regard it to be morally quite justified?'

Evelyn Thomas explains her point of view. These are her own words as reported in the *Observer*:

'When I was found to have breast cancer I had high expectations of the medical profession. Like most patients I believed the doctors observed strict ethical codes. I placed absolute trust in those treating me and assumed that our relationship was based on openness and frankness. I assumed that my treatment was the only option.

'I now know that I assumed too much. Patients with breast cancer presenting themselves to my surgeon in the early 1980s had their treatment determined, without their consent, by computer randomisation. My consultant's role was to diagnose, establish eligibility for entry into clinical trials, withhold information, ensure randomisation and thereafter monitor progress. My rights to have information and to choose, and my responsibility for my own body were denied. My trust was abused. I am both deeply hurt and bitterly disappointed to have been so misused by members of the medical profession.

'In retrospect, the first indication that I was in a trial came a few days after my mastectomy. The mastectomy patient in the next bed had been seen by a counsellor and given helpful information. The counsellor avoided me, and a breast prosthesis was given to me by a male fitter more used to fitting artificial limbs.

'It took several years to obtain confirmation that I had been in a trial. The first trial compared post-operative counselling with no counselling; the availability of counselling was not mentioned to those randomised not to receive it.

'The second trial compared three chemotherapy regimes and no treatment; the regimes were tamoxifen tablets, cyclophosphamide injections and a combination of both. Patients were again randomised – to one of the four choices – without any alternative being offered.

'The administrators at the hospital had confirmed that I was entered into these two trials without my knowledge. Since a trial of lumpectomy versus mastectomy was also in progress at that time I suspect that I may have been in that trial since I was offered no alternative to mastectomy.

'I believe that these trials were wrong for several reasons. At the very least they were unkind. It is unkind not to offer available alternatives to total breast amputation; it is unkind not to offer available counselling to all patients following breast surgery; and it is unkind not to offer to patients an alternative to cyclophosphamide with its side-effect of hair loss that is dreaded.

'Withholding information about the trials may also have invalidated them. It was forgotten that patients, unlike laboratory animals, can move around and communicate

*continues*

*continued*

with each other. Treatments are discussed and unexplained differences discovered. Inevitably these cause worry, and patients may become confused and resentful. Such feelings, and the stress produced, may be the very factors which affect health and well-being . . .

'Secret trials demean patients. By depriving patients of opportunities to make informed choices, doctors appear to assume that we are unintelligent, immature and irresponsible.

'Finally, I believe that such trials are unethical. I agree with the principles laid down in the Nuremburg Code for experiments on humans, which state that "the voluntary consent of the human subject is absolutely essential" and that the person involved "should have sufficient knowledge and comprehension of the elements of the subject matter involved as to enable him to make an understood and enlightened decision".

'Some doctors violate these ethical principles. They argue that patients cannot cope with full knowledge of their disease or uncertainties in its treatment, so that it is kinder to say nothing. Such arguments are wrong, because it is the patient or family who has to cope with an incurable and progressive disease.

'I am not arguing against scientific medical research or randomised clinical trials (RCTs). As a patient I have the most to gain from progress. As a scientist who has herself carried out physiological research on human subjects, obviously I approve of scientific methods in medicine. But RCTs must only be used with the informed consent of the participating patients. If investigators cannot convince patients that each arm of an RCT carries equal chance of risks or benefits then they must respect those patients' decisions not to participate.

'My experience shows that doctors can no longer assume that secrecy in their dealings with patients can remain undetected. Yet once I did start asking questions of my consultant and hospital, the response continued to be secretive. Relevant questions about my treatment have been met with prevarication and half-truths. Approaches to various organisations such as the Community Health Council and the General Medical Council have produced little progress in getting the information, explanation and discussion that I sought. Indeed the only advice offered by the President of the GMC was that I should take legal action – a sorry reflection on the body that has a statutory duty to control the conduct of doctors.

'It is good practice for such trials to be authorised before they start by the hospital's ethical committee, to see whether they are ethically acceptable. The existence of these secret trials therefore raises awkward questions about the committee's role. A letter I received last year from an administrator at the hospital said that informed consent had initially been required for the comparative trial of chemotherapy, but that after a few months the ethical committee had changed its mind. The administrator explained why:

> The reasons for this decision were that the study was being carried out on a National and European level and that other participants on the trial had not felt it appropriate to seek informed consent because of the specifically humane treatment offered in each of the arms of the study. More importantly, the experience nationally and locally was that many patients found it intensely stressful to have to face up to not only consenting to mastectomy but very shortly afterwards to have to consider the true nature of their disease and the uncertainty surrounding its management. The decision-making involved in getting informed consent was considered harmful for the welfare of some patients.

'Such reasons are not adequate to explain why the ethical committee chose to ignore the Nuremburg Code and many subsequent guidelines on the ethical conduct of research.'

Evelyn Thomas's argument was first published anonymously by the *Bulletin of the Institute of Medical Ethics.*

> ## *EXERCISE*
>
> *Either* imagine that you are Doctor Hughes – and that you have read Evelyn's account – and a junior colleague asks you to lead a new research project which requires the diseased patients to be ignorant that they are subjects of research.
>
> *Or* imagine that you are Evelyn and the information has been leaked to you by a sympathetic hospital worker that the research has been proposed, and that it has been put to Dr Hughes that he might like to become involved in it.
>
> Where might Dr Hughes picture himself within the Rings?
>
> Imagine that the doctor and Evelyn both know how to use the Ethical Grid. Imagine a conversation between the two, with the Grid on a table between them. How do you think the discussion would go?

## MISUNDERSTANDING THE IMPORTANCE OF AUTONOMY

The above example shows a doctor placing other values above both the promotion of individual autonomy and respect for choice. There is little question that the motives of researchers in such cases are complex, and often honourable in that the work is directed towards a general increase of human good. But their research is misguided because the importance of autonomy is underestimated.

In the example the researchers place the notions of not causing harm (referring to the stress that might be caused to patients by asking them if they consent to being in a medical experiment), patient welfare (in the sense of not unnecessarily impeding the attempted clinical cure), and the well-being of future patients (who will presumably be helped by advances in the understanding of drug therapies) above that of autonomy (understood in either way). But while it is right to say that autonomy should not always be the primary health care drive, it should not be overridden so lightly. However politically pleasing many might find the view that medicine should work essentially with communities it remains a fact that individuals suffer the disabling problems we call diseases, and that a doctor works most closely with individual patients. Consideration of patient autonomy (in the broadest sense) must always be the starting point for interventions which seek to work for health.

This was obviously not the case in the above example. Three further errors were committed by the medical professor. Briefly, the first was to think of autonomy as a single principle, the second was to commit a category mistake (wrongly supposing that work for health is the natural concomitant of work to counter disease), and the third was to have left Evelyn at a point unnecessarily near the left of the autonomy spectrum when he might – without harm to anybody else – have moved her further to the right. The professor was not working for health in this case. No genuine health work can regard people only as means, even if they are thought to be means towards greater ends.

# THE AUTONOMY FLIP

Before the Autonomy Test is outlined it is important to consider how the notions create and respect autonomy might be ranked in order to guide practical interventions.

## RANKING IDEAS WITHIN AUTONOMY

By attempting to rank these two ideas, an apparently unyielding health care dilemma is again brought to the fore. It is this: to what extent should a person's welfare (autonomy as 'being able to do' – Understanding A) take precedence over a person's wants (autonomy as 'being able to have one's choices' – Understanding B)?

Should welfare ever take precedence over wants? All experienced health carers will be familiar with the frustration of watching a person do something to himself which the health carer thinks is foolish, or tragic, or just 'bloody stupid'. Perhaps the person is eating too much or too little, smoking, drinking, engaging in unprotected sex with several partners or injecting heroin. If the person is indulging in any of these habits, a concerned health carer might well consider that this is not good for him – that it cannot possibly be in his interest even though he thinks it is. Understandably a health worker might think it his task to ensure the person changes his ways.

In such cases there can be a strong temptation for some doctors to be paternalistic – in other words for doctors to give their perception of the person's welfare (often referred to as 'health') a higher priority than his choice.

Such a policy assumes this ranking of the two notions of autonomy:

FIRST: CREATE AUTONOMY

SECOND: RESPECT AUTONOMY

The expression create autonomy refers to basic work to enable a person (Understanding A), to work to provide adequate conditions of welfare – conditions for a way of life where a person is able to realise fulfilling possibilities. For instance, educating a person about the effect of medication on her body, and ensuring that an extremely stressed person takes a rest, are both actions which would qualify as work to create autonomy.

Create autonomy ought to take precedence over respect autonomy when a person clearly faces disabling problems, and makes no objection to the health worker addressing these problems. However, at a point which varies – dependent upon circumstances and the individuals concerned – the two notions 'flip over' like this:

FIRST: RESPECT AUTONOMY

SECOND: CREATE AUTONOMY

The ultimate aim of work to create autonomy is to move a person to a position where she is so unfettered that she is able to exercise an informed choice about what she would like, and be able to get it. It should be self-evident that:

Education for health is work for wholeness. It is not just to do with physical functioning, it is at least equally to do with the mental life of a person . . . work for health in its full and proper sense is work towards laying the foundations for full human flourishing.[1]

Human beings are distinguished from most animals by our facility to think – to reflect, to introspect, to plan our actions. Not to pay particular attention to this human asset when working for health is absurd.

The central ethical problem in health care occurs when a carer wants to carry on creating autonomy (as welfare) while the subject believes he has reached a level of autonomy sufficient to permit a reasoned choice, and wants his autonomy respected. This may mean that the subject wishes to have further autonomy created, but in a way unacceptable to the health worker.

Consider a case from practice. Take the example of a person said to be 'abusing heroin'. While create autonomy is ranked first, the health worker can justifiably seek to push the person to the right of the spectrum. So, if the drug taker seeks help whilst intoxicated the health worker might offer facilities for treatment, might educate about the risks of heroin injection, might counsel, might review the person's life circumstances to see if a changed life-style might be preferable (and possible) as an alternative to heroin-taking, might show the safest ways of injecting, and might argue for whatever point of view she believes in (so long as she does not present this as the only worthwhile possibility, so long as she does not take advantage of the person's vulnerability to put forward propaganda).

However, once the autonomy flip has occurred work to create autonomy can continue but must always be implemented so as to take the fullest possible account of the wishes of the subject of health care. So, if the drug taker says something to this effect, 'I have listened to all you have to say, I have learnt from you, but I do not wish to stop my habit, and I do not wish you to try to make me stop anymore', and it is clear that he has the capacity to understand and has made an informed choice, then this wish must be respected.

Of course the duty to respect autonomy is not absolute in all cases. For instance, it is inappropriate if a parent insists 'I wish to continue inflicting unnecessary suffering on my children'. Autonomy ought not be respected if a person's choice will deliberately harm others, and the harm is avoidable. Equally, it might be the case that a health worker has to take wider considerations into account, that to respect individual autonomy in all cases might be to go against what might loosely be described as the 'public interest' (perhaps if the doctor were not to report a chronic epileptic patient seen driving a car).

Neither is it an implication of a commitment to respect autonomy that whatever a person wishes should be provided. It does not follow that because a patient wants ampoules of heroin on prescription a doctor has a duty to oblige. But what is implied is that once choice is possible, once the human faculty of reason is present, then the doctor should not positively prevent this choice unless respecting the wish would cause harm to others, or seriously undermine the subject's welfare and the subject does not recognise this.

# THE AUTONOMY TEST

The Autonomy Test applies only to health care and only to individuals.

In the arena of urgent practice, images and models may seem nothing more than a diversion from reality. Such decision-making tools require time to think through and apply, and this time is not available to most health workers. If Paradigm Y is not to remain an optimistic hope something immediately applicable is needed.

On many occasions in health care decisions have to be made quickly, even though there are no simple rules available. What is required in these circumstances is a 'litmus test', a speedy way of obtaining a provisional indication whether a proposed course of action ought to go ahead or not, or if it ought to be modified.

Although many health care decisions are perennially debatable, some policies are clearly wrong. The Autonomy Test is of most value in its ability to help expose these cases. It also helps to clarify options for creative progress by focusing on practical ways of moving a person to the right of the autonomy spectrum.

## WHAT IS THE AUTONOMY TEST?

The Autonomy Test is a basic means of checking the appropriateness of plans, and of 'brainstorming' for better possibilities for care. However, the Autonomy Test is also a result of a systematic account of the nature of health, and to use it is to concede many implicit assumptions.

---

**The Autonomy Test – Annotated**

The Autonomy Test consists of a number of simple questions, and requires the health worker simply to list various possibilities.

ONE

*Will physical or mental autonomy not be increased when it might have been? Will it be diminished in any way?*

This is a very demanding question. Only rarely in the context of medical interventions will it be possible honestly to answer NO to this question. It is very strict. The question requires that if a drug is prescribed with 'side effects' which diminish, or a person has to stay in hospital, then the response must at this stage be YES. If there is doubt about whether or not an intervention is one which acts to diminish then, if possible, seek the opinion of the subject.

If the answer is genuinely NO then go to SIX. If the answer is YES, or if there is any possibility that it might be YES because a factor has been overlooked, then go to TWO.

*continues*

---

_ continued _

TWO

*List the way(s) in which autonomy will be increased and the way(s) in which autonomy will be diminished by the proposed action:*

**Increases in Autonomy**          **Diminishings of Autonomy**

Note: At this point it is inevitable that there will be disagreement about what things count as increases (enablings) and what as decreases of autonomy (diminishings). It is likely that there will be particular debate over the question of long-term and short-term autonomy. Some will take the view that although autonomy (either in the sense of being able to have wishes fulfilled, or in the sense of being able to move unfettered) is diminished in the short term, this is justified by the probable long-term increase. (This position is sometimes asserted when people are detained – in their perceived best interests – under Mental Health Acts.)

THREE

*Are each of these diminishings absolutely necessary?*

If NO, then STOP

Reconsider the proposed action. Consider a fresh policy.

If YES, then go to

FOUR

*Will these diminishings have the effect of increasing the autonomy of the patient (according to either Understanding A or B) in the future?*

If NO, then STOP. Reconsider the proposed action. Consider a policy which might work for health instead.

If YES, then go to

FIVE

*Are the patient's reasoned wishes being overridden?*

If NO, and the intent is to move the person to the right of the autonomy spectrum as soon as possible, then proceed to SIX.

If YES, then either STOP – a *category mistake* will be committed if disease is challenged at the expense of human choice – or show how this overriding of reasoned wants can be justified in another way. Possible justifications might include:

_ continues _

— *continued* —

1. The individual's wishes will harm me or others unnecessarily.
2. The individual is reasoning erroneously – he may be thinking illogically – he may be deriving false conclusions, or he may have false beliefs (but, if so, then an attempt must be made to move him as soon as possible to the point where the *autonomy flip* can occur).

Note: At this point in the Autonomy Test it is very important to bear in mind the distinction between physical autonomy – the freedom that a person has to live without physical obstruction – and mental autonomy – the freedom that a person has to make decisions and act on them. It is usual for short-term physical autonomy to be decreased in health care in order to increase long-term physical autonomy – restraining an arm in a sling, or prescribing drugs which cause drowsiness in order to cure infections, or injuring a person during surgery: all these are reductions in short-term physical mobility. So long as these diminishings are not imposed against a person's wishes, they are not problematic. But here the insidiousness of the category mistake becomes truly apparent. Although it is a genuine mistake which implies no intent to harm, the mistake can be dangerous. It is one thing to stop a broken leg moving by slapping plaster of paris around it, yet quite another to prevent a person acting on her choice to drink 'too much' or to have 'too many boyfriends', by classifying her as ill and administering long-lasting tranquillisers. The reduction of mental autonomy, even in the short term with the goal of promoting long-term gain, is far harder to justify in the case of any rational person (whether child or adult) who can understand the implications of what she proposes to do.

Justifications have been attempted, but they smack of the miserliness of spirit – just as a financial miser will be forever saving, waiting just a little longer until he spends. For example, it has been argued that breaking a confidence (in other words not respecting a person's choice) is justified so long as this results in greater autonomy for that person in the long term. But it is hard to see the purpose of this. If the person is in a position to choose, then he should be permitted this. Otherwise, on the next occasion that the person with the power to deny choice disagrees with that choice, she will be able to justify its denial by saying that the patient is not yet autonomous enough.

What such an argument basically says is this: although you do have the capacity to choose for yourself, either you are making the wrong choice deliberately, or you cannot see that by choosing this choice you are shutting a great many doors that would otherwise be open to you. Thus, for the sake of your future capacity to choose – which should be as great as possible – I override your present capacity – and I do it for your sake.

Naturally many kind and experienced people do pursue policies such as this with those they feel could benefit from their 'hidden' support. However, it is always open to such well-meaning closet paternalists to explain in the fullest possible terms why they believe that the other person is making a mistake. There is the danger that since there is no theoretical cut-off point – no binding rule to tell the paternalist when he has gone too far, or continued for too long – that he will, using exactly the same justification time and time again, continue to override personal choice.

— *continues* —

*continued*

The Autonomy Test is clear on this. To satisfy the Autonomy Test the flip should occur just as soon as the person can weigh up the problem, review the options, and assess the implications. A free society does not wait until some ideal inspired moment – people must be free to make mistakes.

## SIX

*Consider the list of the ways in which autonomy might be increased (the ways in which latent enhancing human potentials might be made actual). Decide, if at all possible in partnership with the patient, the order of priority in which this list of possible potentials might be achieved.*

*Weigh these against any potential costs.*

## SEVEN

*Once decided and agreed – initiate proposed action.*

---

### The Autonomy Test – Unannotated

## ONE

*Will physical or mental autonomy not be increased when it might have been? Will it be diminished in any way?*

If the answer is genuinely NO, then go to SIX. If the answer is YES, or if there is any possibility that it might be YES because a factor has been overlooked, then go to TWO.

## TWO

*List the way(s) in which autonomy will be increased and the way(s) in which autonomy will be diminished by the proposed action:*

**Increases in Autonomy**          **Diminishings of Autonomy**

## THREE

*Are each of these diminishings absolutely necessary?*

If NO then STOP. Reconsider the proposed action. Consider a fresh policy.

If YES, then go to

## FOUR

*Will these diminishings have the effect of increasing the autonomy (according to either Understanding A or B) of the patient in the future?*

If NO then STOP. Reconsider the proposed action. Consider a policy which might work for health.

*continues*

*continued*

If YES then go to

FIVE

*Are the patient's reasoned wishes being overridden?*

If NO, and the intent is to move the person to the right of the autonomy spectrum as soon as possible, then proceed to SIX.

If YES, then either STOP – the *category mistake* will be committed if disease is challenged at the expense of human choice – show how this overriding of reasoned wants can be justified in another way. Go to SIX.

SIX

*Consider the list of the ways in which autonomy might be increased (the ways in which latent enhancing human potentials might be made actual). Decide, if at all possible in partnership with the patient, the order of priority in which this list of possible potentials might be achieved.*

*Weigh these against any potential costs.*

SEVEN

*Once decided and agreed – initiate proposed action.*

## APPLYING THE AUTONOMY TEST

Although the Autonomy Test is crude and open to interpretation, it is nevertheless a guideline that health workers might choose to adopt. It is enlightening to apply the test to various cases in real life. This will usually give clear answers. It is not necessary to go into detailed ethical analysis of most of these cases since the Autonomy Test makes no claim to depth – it is a litmus test, a traffic light: Should I stop or should I go? For instance, if Carole's case (see p. 187) is put to the Autonomy Test there is a swift result.

### The Test Applied – Carole

ONE

*Will physical or mental autonomy not be increased when it might have been? Will it be diminished in any way?*

**Answer**   Yes, unequivocally. Carole is an intelligent and able girl, yet she does not have enough information about her diagnosis and her treatment. Perhaps even more importantly no work is being done to help her *picture* what is happening to her, to help her conceive of the set of unfortunate circumstances which currently surround her – to help her map out her world. Carole desperately needs to recognise that all her problems are not her fault, that failure is just one map out of several possibilities, and that all maps have routes into each other – we can and will all fail at some things.

.

*continues*

*continued*

TWO

*List the way(s) in which autonomy will be increased and the way(s) in which autonomy will be diminished by the proposed action.*

| Increases in Autonomy | Diminishings of Autonomy |
|---|---|
| | (Note: not increasing autonomy where it would be possible to do so is taken to be diminishing) |
| Possible alleviation of psychotic symptoms | Things done to Carole without her understanding |
| | Family not involved in any therapy |
| | No counselling – no picturing for Carole |
| | No attempt to help Carole to find a purpose in her life |

THREE

*Are each of these diminishings absolutely necessary?*

**Answer**   No. Reconsider the proposed action. Consider a fresh policy.

---

## *EXERCISE*

Apply the Autonomy Test to the example highlighted by Evelyn Thomas, outlined earlier on pp. 188–190. Address this proposal: Dr Hughes wants to carry out an identical research programme on human subjects. Consider your response with reference to one of the potential subjects, Pauline Johnson.

## THE LIMITATION OF THE AUTONOMY TEST

There is much that the Autonomy Test cannot do. There are many cases where what counts as an increase or decrease in autonomy is too open to interpretation for the test to be decisive. To resolve such cases more extensive ethical analysis is necessary, although the Autonomy Test will hardly ever be entirely redundant.

For instance, consider the following difficult case:

LAW REPORT

### Sterilisation of mental patient not unlawful

A sterilisation operation on a mentally disabled adult patient is not unlawful by reason only of the patient's inability to consent if it is carried out in the best interests of the patient.

*The facts*

F., who was born in 1953, has the verbal capacity of a two year old and the general mental capacity of a four to five year old. She has been a voluntary inpatient at a hospital since 1967, where she has formed a sexual relationship with a male mental patient. The evidence was that she had physical enjoyment from sexual intercourse with him and that she was not being sexually molested.

F. has the fertility of any other woman of her age, and her mother applied for a declaration that it would be lawful for F. to be sterilised, notwithstanding that she was incapable of consenting. Mr Justice Scott-Baker granted the declaration (Guardian Law Report 3 December 1988). The Official Solicitor, who was given leave to intervene, appealed.

*The decision*

Lord Donaldson referred to the case of Re B[1988]AC199 in which the House of Lords held that in the case of a mentally handicapped minor the court could, acting in its wardship jurisdiction, consent to the sterilisation of the minor if it was in her best interests. This raised the stark issue of whether the law treated adults who suffered from a disability differently, and on one view less favourably, than it treated children suffering from a similar disability. In the absence of consent all, or almost all, medical and surgical treatment of an adult is unlawful, however beneficial such treatment might be.

F.'s disability was such that she would never be mentally competent to appreciate the issues involved and to consent to sterilisation or to any medical treatment. The court had no power either under the *parens patriae* jurisdiction or under any statutory jurisdiction to dispense with F.'s consent or to give consent on her behalf.

The common law right of body inviolability save with consent was subject to two exceptions: first, emergency medical treatment, and second, physical contacts which are inevitable or at least are a usual feature of everyday life, such as the jostling on public transport, or generally acceptable standards of conduct. A doctor faced with an unconscious accident patient is lawfully entitled and probably bound to carry out such treatment as is necessary to safeguard the patient's life and health, although the patient is in no position to consent.

It would therefore not be surprising if the common law rule were subject to a further qualification in relation to those who by reason of disability are unable to consent. There is a clear and logical connection between the position of an adult who through an accident is temporarily deprived of the power of consent – the emergency treatment case – and the case of an adult who through permanent disability is equally unable to consent. The difference is largely, although not entirely, one of scale.

But the law should not regard adults as permanent emergency cases. In an emergency a doctor had little time but in this case the doctor had more time, and far more was required of him.

The test which the court did, and the reasonable adult should, apply was, 'what course of action is best calculated to promote my true welfare and interests'. What constituted true welfare and interests often gave rise to very difficult questions, but that did not affect the validity of the test . . .

Lord Justice Neill said the answer lay in considering the public interest. Provided that the operation was necessary within properly defined limits and appropriate safeguards were prescribed, there was no reason in principle why a patient who could not give consent should be deprived of the right to receive the treatment required.

'Necessary' in that context meant that which a general body of medical opinion in the particular specialty would consider to be in the best interests of the patient in order to maintain his health and secure his well-being. Unanimity was not required, but it should be possible to say of an operation which was necessary in the relevant sense that it would be unreasonable in the opinion of most experts in the field not to make the operation available to the patient.

Lord Justice Butler-Sloss concurred.

The appeal was dismissed, and leave was granted to appeal to the House of Lords.[83]

The problem for the Autonomy Test in these circumstances is that the autonomy flip can never occur. F. will never be able to have a sufficient level of autonomy created for her to enable her to consider her situation, and to express a wish.

The judges decided to apply a 'best interests test', but what one person might consider to be in her 'best interests', another might not. For example, a critic of the judgement argued:

> There are a number of deeply disturbing features about this case. It is not clear that the court had the jurisdiction to make the order that it did. And it is not clear that the order made was legally correct. To equate the sterilisation operation, as the judge did, with the extraction of a tooth, the repair of a hernia or the administration of an injection, fails to recognise the enormity of the invasion and injury which the proposed sterilisation represents. It fails to distinguish between the obvious therapeutic advantages in the supposed analogies and the dubious benefits which sterilisation offers. And it fails to acknowledge that sterilisation involves major abdominal surgery requiring general anaesthesia . . .
>
> As troubling, however, are the assumptions being made about the sexuality of women with a mental handicap, the risks to which pregnancy exposes them, and the response of courts to the interests of what the judge in one place calls 'mental defectives'.[84]

For the judges and the author of this quote the list of increases and diminishings is not the same. A judgement has to be made about who gives the most appropriate list in regard to the creation of F.'s autonomy, and this is not finally decidable. An analysis deeper than the Autonomy Test is required for this, but at least the Autonomy Test offers guidance in setting limits, and compels the listing of possibilities.

Clearly there is a difficulty with the ranking of dwarfings. Since a dwarfing must be avoided, unless to do it will prevent a worse dwarfing, it must be possible to state in general terms how one thing is worse than another. But how can subjective preferences be assessed in an objective way? Often this cannot be done – people's preferences are not the same. In such cases, the only way forward is to find out, in individual context, what the person wants. This is where the autonomy flip is useful – and where one must respect the liberty of other people. Where the autonomy flip cannot occur, great care must be taken that clearly avoidable dwarfings do not happen – and this judgement must rest on a deeper analysis and weighing of the potential and probable harms.

## EXERCISE

Re-read **The Operation** in the Introduction pp. 12–19. Imagine that you are the surgeon (a) during the initial consultation and (b) as he meets the patient on the morning of the operation. Use the Autonomy Test and base a moral policy on its results.

## RESPECT AUTONOMY (brief explanation)

The requirement to respect autonomy is also part of the core rationale of health work (the blue boxes), but as we have seen is significantly different from the necessity to create autonomy. The creation of autonomy requires the provision of the physical and mental wherewithal for enhanced movement in life, whereas respecting autonomy requires that the person's chosen direction should be respected, whether or not the health worker approves of it.

This idea is bedevilled with controversy. Many of the really hard cases in medical ethics hinge upon whether or not 'respect autonomy' should be invoked. Some of these controversies can be settled with intelligent use of the grid, but there are no binding guidelines about how far personal (or group) autonomy ought to be respected. A strong (though not immutable) reason not to respect autonomy arises when the autonomous decision will harm other people. Beyond this, the issues must be resolved by personal judgement and comprehensive and appropriate moral reasoning.

## RESPECT PERSONS EQUALLY

The requirement to respect persons equally when working for health follows from the requirement to create and respect autonomy in everyone. We regard people as valuable not only because of what each can do, but because of what each is. The cardinal aspects of personhood – being able to value one's life and having the potential for future choices – are shared equally by all persons.

The extent to which the box 'respect persons equally' should be employed is a matter of judgement. However, as with the other blue boxes, if this box is to be superseded firmly convincing reasons are required. If persons are not respected equally, perhaps because resources are scarce, then this is discrimination between beings who are fundamentally equal. If such discrimination is condoned by a health service for unjustifiable reasons then there are dangerous implications for that society as a whole. If it is all right for a health service to discriminate on grounds of age, race and economic worth, then other social institutions have *carte blanche* to do the same.

## SERVE NEEDS FIRST

This element of the core provides a grounding for the other three. It gains its authority firstly from the fact that a true health service must – before any other task – provide for the basic needs of all it seeks to serve, and secondly from an underpinning association between work for health and justice as fairness. Since those who have made a commitment to work for health are obliged to create autonomy and treat persons with equal respect it follows that they must also want to ensure that everyone's basic needs are met. So, if there are people who have no shelter, or no food, or no purpose in life, or a very limited general education, while in the same society there are people whose material wants are being over-fulfilled then this is a system in which full health is not being achieved. It is a system in which there is a lower degree of morality than there otherwise might be.

All human beings have needs that are part of a shared human condition. Though they are never absolute,[58] they may be said to be factual. Rights vary over history and between contexts, and although it is argued by some that through hard work some people deserve more benefits in life than those who do not work so hard, it seems fundamentally unjust for such rewards to be enjoyed at the expense of basic human needs (though it must be admitted that despite millenia of philosophical labour, no one has yet succeeded in demonstrating that this is *necessarily* so).[5]

But what is so important about medicine and health work is that this principle has so often been followed in practice. In wartime medics do not (or should not if they are health workers) treat only the wounded from their army, and medical treatment is commonly offered to criminals regardless of what crime they have committed. Within health work it seems there is an elemental humanising principle at work. While some pains and some diseases may be socially caused and avoidable, many are not. A person unlucky enough to become unwell needs help and needs it unconditionally. When it is so given it is a pure moral donation – a giving based on sympathy and a desire to create better possibilities for others. By contrast, if a hospital turns away one person with a broken leg whilst admitting another, on the ground that the first person is a bank robber and the second a bank manager, health workers have no difficulty in recognising that the action of the hospital is morally superficial.

# IN SUMMARY

## A REVIEW

### Why Are the Blue Boxes Core?

#### The Devil's Advocate Speaks Again

> All that is going on in this writing about health and ethics is a cleverish word game based on a set of improvable assumptions that you take for granted. You have decided what health is, and now, by the use of sophistry more than anything else, you attempt to deceive us into thinking that you are uncovering truths. But you are doing nothing of the sort. You are not a detective, you are an inventor. In order to defeat your position one need only refuse to accept your assumptions and make alternative ones instead – perhaps premises more acceptable to a person of a different political persuasion. For instance, one might just as well include these (or any other) boxes within the core 'health rationale': manipulate clients, create dependency, discriminate between individuals according to their social worth, and act to provide a service for those who, through their own efforts, can pay for it, and do so before you pay any attention to the worthless needy.

Harsh words, but they are from an exasperating devil's advocate who has not understood the argument of this book (and companion texts).[1,5] The point of these works is to provide a firm theoretical footing for a true health service, a health service which aims as its first priority to increase the degree of morality in the world through the interventions made in the name of health. It is undeniable that assumptions about

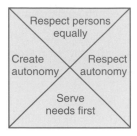

**Figure 26**   The blue boxes

what a 'true health service' is are just that – assumptions. They are preferences and cannot be empirically shown to define work for health. But on the other hand there is a rich and varied set of reasons behind them. These reasons are connected as threads in a tapestry. They begin and end in different places, but link together to present a compelling picture. Some of the threads the devil's advocate should see stitched together are:

1. It has been shown that work for health has a common factor – namely the removal of obstacles to people's biological and intellectual potentials.
2. The associated ideas of 'enablement', 'personhood', and 'enhancing potential' are (a) richer, more coherent and logically sound than the speculative alternatives of the advocate and (b) more likely to produce benefits that can be shared by all than any other option.
3. There is a clear relationship between ethics and health, demonstrated in these pages and elsewhere.
4. Certain actions can be considered to be immoral because they dwarf gratuitously. Those features vulnerable to the most serious dwarfing are precisely those which provide the basis for the equal treatment of persons.
5. The existing rationale of health work – in theory and in practice – cannot be ignored. Although things could be better and priorities reassessed, study of present health work practice shows that the principles outlined in the blue layer are already those that inspire much work in the name of health. The seeds of Paradigm Y are already sown in Paradigm X.
6. The practical consequences of the devil's advocate's idea are dreadful. How could a health service be organised according to these principles? Such a service would not be a legitimate health service because although it would seek to remove some obstacles to some potentials it would not do for all people equally, and some of the potentials – if achieved – would be debilitating, not enhancing.

Bear firmly in mind, before moving on, that in all but the most exceptional cases at least one blue box should be used during deliberations. A decision to ignore all four needs a massive justification. It is usually impossible to work for health without invoking a blue box.

## THE RED LAYER

This level of the grid focuses on duties and motive. The boxes included are illustrated in Figure 27.

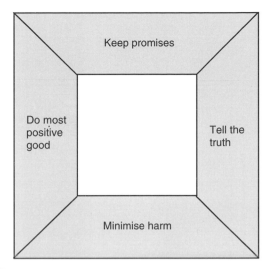

**Figure 27**   The red boxes

## WHAT IS THE SIGNIFICANCE OF THIS LAYER?

The red layer corresponds with deontological outlooks, and contrasts with the green, consequentialist layer. It is meant to encourage consideration of obligations other than those immediately implied by a commitment to health work. The duties shown are not the only ones possible (*not killing, not causing unnecessary pain, being compassionate*, and *taking due care* are some of the alternatives) but are probably the most commonly recognised amongst health workers. Nor are these duties meant to be binding. They should never be dispensed with casually, but from time to time situations will occur where it is better that they are temporarily disregarded and excluded from use. However, when thinking about health work interventions it is important to bring moral obligations to mind and if one, more, or even all are to be disregarded then very good reasons must be advanced in justification.

## THE GREEN LAYER

The green layer divides consequentialism into four key aspects in order to focus attention on outcomes of proposed interventions, and to encourage moral reasoners to clarify their priorities. Ethical confusions commonly arise between health professionals because they have failed to agree who 'the patient is'. It is often assumed that one's own target of concern is the same as everyone else's, when this is not so. In the same case a nurse may be seeking to maximise benefit for an individual, a social worker may see the family as the unit of care, a doctor may want to maximise benefit for all her patients, and so on. If these matters are not spelt out needless tensions can be created. Attention to the green layer will promote reflection about whether benefit (which must also be discussed and specified in advance) should be increased for humanity as a whole, for a particular group (perhaps a disadvantaged group such as the

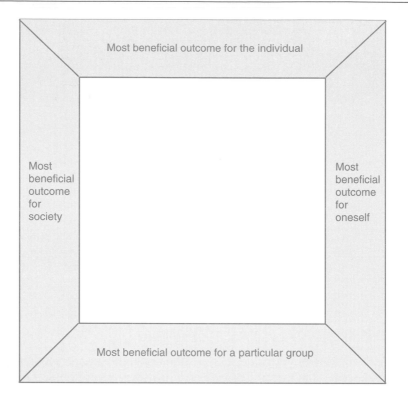

**Figure 28**    The green boxes

handicapped, members of the black community, people living in a particular housing estate), for an individual, or for the agent herself.

As with the other layers – and indeed the whole Grid – nothing is clear-cut. It may be that all the boxes of the green layer can be brought into play, or that only some can be used while others lie redundant, or it may be that a box will have to be chosen at the expense of other boxes.

For example, when considering an intervention it might be concluded that the interests of a particular group might have to be sacrificed in order to bring about an increase in social good. So it might be that renal physicians and patient groups get together to decide on the best use of scarce dialysis machines and kidneys, and in so doing agree a ranking of potential beneficiaries from 'essential' to 'inappropriate'. As they do this they will inevitably arbitrate in favour of the youngest and strongest recipients – placing the interests of a particular group (the oldest and sickest) as a lower priority.

But this is not necessarily the fairest or most morally desirable decision, and the green layer should be used only in conjunction with the grid as a whole.

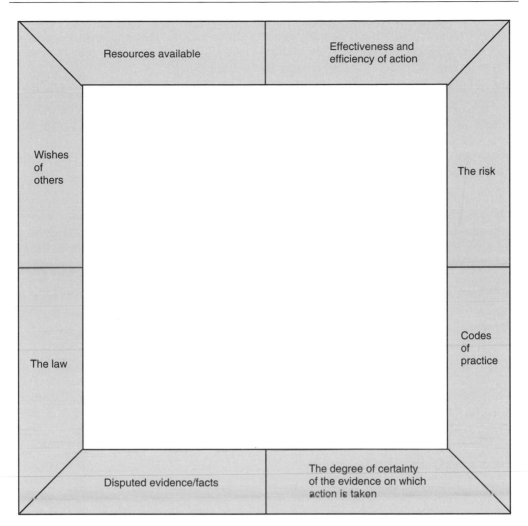

**Figure 29**   The black boxes

## THE BLACK LAYER

The black layer is of great importance, yet includes factors often given insufficient attention by moral philosophers. The black layer is the level of external considerations. In many cases, in the hard world we live in, the black layer contains the most important factors. For instance, it may be that a person's legal right – say to receive advice or treatment – effectively takes any decision out of the hands of the health worker.

Ethics is not only a matter of deciding on principles, considering duties, and reflecting on likely outcomes in the abstract. Ethical intervention takes place in a perpetually uncertain world of limitations. Although it has been shown that law and morality do not necessarily correspond, existing law will have a clear part to play in some deliberations. Professional codes of practice, although sometimes vague and imprecise, may have a bearing on certain interventions, and it is for the health worker to decide when, if ever, these codes provide sufficient advice.

It is also necessary to assess an intervention's degree of risk, in whichever of many possible senses of risk are most relevant. Will physical harm occur? Will there be emotional damage? Is there a danger that an unfortunate precedent will be set? Is there a chance that the proposed intervention will produce unintended consequences? There is an associated demand on the Grid user to try to ensure that whatever intervention made is carried out with maximum efficiency and effectiveness.

It is also necessary to consider the degree of certainty of the evidence on which the action is to be taken, and to take account of those facts of the matter that are clear and undisputed. Not to do so would, by any standard, be foolish. Moreover, it is important not only to 'respect people' in the abstract, but to ascertain what their wishes are in practice. Since most professional health workers are in a position of some power and status, many clients may be overawed and have decisions imposed on them, even if the imposition is unwitting. Health workers should in every case try to clarify the wishes of those they are trying to help, and of those other people who care for them and are affected by what happens to them, and should try to help them conceive of their position and choices as plainly and accurately as possible.

Finally, there is an abiding responsibility (implied by the Grid as a whole) on anyone who intervenes in the life of another person to be able to justify all actions by reference to the evidence. Any person who has reasoned morally in a proper fashion will be in an excellent position to do this.

## THE LIMIT TO THE GRID

The limit to the Grid is straightforward. It can be used properly only by those who honestly seek to enable people's enhancing potentials. The Ethical Grid can be used legitimately only by those who are consistently opposed to dwarfing, and devoted to the fight against it.

The Grid can be used as it is supposed to be only by people who have made a commitment to work for health, and are seeking to do so with integrity. If it is used insincerely, if the Grid is employed cynically – merely in order to further personal goals, for instance – then this is not a moral use, even though the outcomes might sometimes be the same as those which result from sincere use.

## A CLAIM FOR THE GRID, AND WHAT IT CANNOT DO

The Ethical Grid is a tool, and nothing more than that. Like a hammer or a screwdriver used competently, it can help make certain tasks easier, but it cannot direct the tasks, nor can it help decide which tasks are the most important. The Grid can enhance deliberation – it can throw light into unseen corners and can suggest new avenues of

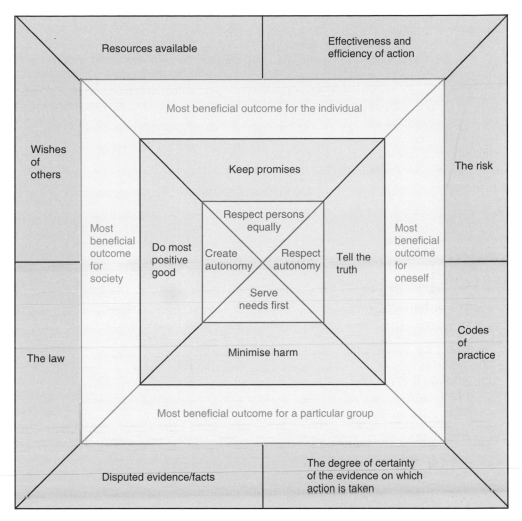

**Figure 30**    The Ethical Grid

thought – but it is not a substitute for personal judgement. True moral reasoning is an essentially human activity which touches sensitive nerves and exposes emotional frailty. Responsibility lies with the user, not the Grid.

# CHAPTER ELEVEN

# The Use of the Ethical Grid

## HOW TO USE THE ETHICAL GRID

Various uses of the Ethical Grid are possible.[85] Which method to adopt is up to the user, though the following approach is highly recommended.

### IN GENERAL

It is recommended that the Ethical Grid be brought into play at every opportunity (at first even when matters of health are not of central concern). When reading newspapers, watching television documentaries, reading literature, when considering friends' life problems, or when considering one's own responses to difficult situations, it is helpful to practise with the Grid to understand its possibilities and limitations.

### IN PRACTICE

1. Consider the issue without reference to the Grid. Clarify the issue by identifying key aspects. Attempt to list the pros and cons of the various options for action. Try to imagine possible ramifications. Arrive at an initial position about what ought to be done.

   Though it is not a requirement, health workers may find the Rings of Uncertainty (see Chapter 9) helpful in this – especially in complicated cases.
2. Express a *specific question* or state a *clear hypothesis*.

   This is essential to productive use of the Grid – a vaguely focused investigation will fail. The best method is to form a hypothesis – I should do X – based on one's post-clarification response, and then try to show what's wrong with it by use of the Grid. Most users find this psychologically difficult, preferring to search the Grid for 'evidence' to 'confirm' their initial view. But this is a poor use. Given so many levels and aspects it is not difficult to find the reasons one wants. However, the point of the Grid is to enable genuine exploration of both policy and motivation – so it is better to find a way to counter one's biases. If it is found too hard to argue against a favoured hypothesis then the Grid should be surveyed in the company of people likely to disagree.

   If the Grid is used in such a group – and it is an ideal vehicle for case conferences and team meetings – it is important to appoint an independent chairperson to take notes, spot inconsistencies, resolve disputes, obtain further evidence, clarify philosophical points and keep the group focused on the Grid's categories. Though this may seem a tall order at first, once the Grid has been used by the same group just a few times it should be possible to rotate the Chair, and so to build up expertise in all members.

The Grid is meant to make moral reasoning explicit. Its most successful use, therefore, is when everyone with an interest in a problem is involved in decision-making. Explicit moral reasoning is public moral reasoning. This means that wherever possible patients – and their supporters if they wish – should be able to use the Grid with other team members. To decide not to involve patients is itself a moral matter, and requires strong justification.

Using the Grid this way will be time-consuming and will require health workers to educate patients to a greater extent than they normally would. However, this is precisely what health workers should be doing anyway – to say it is too difficult, or gets in the way of clinical priorities, or confuses patients, or is only suitable for a certain kind of patient are all Paradigm X excuses. It would not, for instance, be impossibly difficult to prepare a pamphlet for patients on 'Moral Issues Which May Face You and Your Carers', and explain how to make use of the Grid in this.

3. Consider the Grid. Either start at the outside and work in (this is the method preferred by most practically disposed people) or begin with the layer which feels most significant. Often a colour or box will seem to leap out as an obvious place to start.

4. Consider all other levels of the Grid. Select – after appropriate weighing and balancing – those boxes which appear to offer the best solution (those which seem most likely to create health – to produce the highest degree of morality).

   It is not necessary to consider every box. Their importance varies with each context, and sometimes some are of no relevance. However, it is recommended that novice users do reflect on every box – until they become familiar with the Grid procedure.

5. Arrange the boxes 'over' (see Introduction, pp. 2–4) the dilemma to check how the solution looks. If the Grid and associated tools have been used well then the problem will have been thoroughly clarified, clear questions and/or hypotheses will have been tested, a range of factors (philosophical, evidential and moral) will have been considered, the process will have been open, it will have been recorded (in writing or on tape), one or more boxes will have been selected – and a reasoned decision will have been made.

## TWO CASE STUDIES CONSIDERED WITH THE USE OF THE ETHICAL GRID

### I.   TEACHING OR CARING: MICHAEL AND CAROLINE

Recall Michael, the empathic health visitor assigned an elderly widow as part of his training (pp. 56–57). Although Caroline did not need nursing Michael visited her for eight months, and the two became friends. Both were benefiting from the friendship.

When Michael qualified his supervisor assigned him a different case load, even though he was still operating the same area. She explained that Caroline's circumstances did not merit the services of a busy, qualified health visitor, and that the old lady had really been useful only as part of Michael's learning experience. Michael accepted this with great reluctance, but responded that he would, in this case, continue to visit Caroline in a private capacity. But his supervisor forbade even this, threatening that it would be a 'very unprofessional' thing to do.

## Different Thinking

### Dennis' Thoughts

Two health workers have reviewed the case and arrived at these initial stances.

Dennis feels there is something profoundly wrong about the supervisor's treatment of the pair. It seems to him that Michael and Caroline, in their own ways, both wish to enable each other – not solely as a means of furthering their own self-interests, but in a way that respects the individuality of the other. Dennis suspects the supervisor has a hidden motive. Perhaps she feels that Michael's enthusiastic approach to his work – and his obvious success – pose a threat to her authority, and so she needs to undermine him.

Dennis thinks the following proposal will create the highest degree of morality. Since two people will benefit Michael should ignore the wishes of his supervisor and continue to visit Caroline while at the same time performing a responsible and caring role with his new case load. (Note that Dennis has chosen to focus on Michael's options for action since he sees him as the central character. His *specific question* was 'Should Michael continue to visit Caroline?' He might have converted this to the hypothesis: Michael should continue to visit Caroline.)

### Mary's Thoughts

Mary feels there is something too impulsive about Michael's behaviour, and she also has a 'gut feeling' that the overall interests of Michael's colleagues will not be served by the supervisor approving of Michael's request, or by her turning a blind eye to his visits.

Mary sees Michael and Caroline as mavericks, rebels who unintentionally threaten to disrupt the smooth running of a system which – in the way it operates at present, by rules, codes, hierarchies, and established principles – works to serve the best interests of the community as a whole.

Mary reckons the supervisor is the central character. She thinks the most ethical intervention the supervisor can make is to insist, if necessary in the strongest terms, that Michael obeys her request as behoves a professional.

Mary does not regard this as callous. She takes Michael's feelings (and future as a good health visitor) fully into account – she considers that the supervisor's 'hard line' is in Michael's best interest. The supervisor should, in addition to her reprimand, see to it that Michael receives proper counselling, in-service training, and even career guidance if he cannot bring himself to accept the decision.

Mary has concluded that Caroline is perfectly capable of looking after herself, and should not be a burden on public funds. She believes that neither the public's nor Caroline's interests will be best served by her continuing a relationship that began, and should have remained, as one between health visitor and client. In Mary's opinion prolonging the relationship will be good for neither Caroline nor Michael, neither will it benefit Michael's other clients since it could interfere with his professional responsibilities toward clients in genuine need.

# THE GRID IN USE

Now that the key factors have been listed by the health workers concerned the Grid can be brought into service. It may be that it will confirm an initial position, lending it substance and intellectual credibility, or maybe it will lead to a change of mind. Whatever the case, the Grid should be useful.

## A Possible Use of the Grid by Mary

Mary, who is honestly seeking to liberate as many enhancing potentials as possible, is drawn immediately to the green layer of the grid. After due reflection on the key factors of the case (which she has listed as 'professional responsibility', 'the public interest', 'respect for authority', and 'the maintenance of codes of practice') she believes the long-term consequences of the supervisor's intervention should be the overriding consideration. She feels that if the supervisor insists on obedience then the consequences for all concerned will be better – Michael especially will benefit – and that the consequences for society as a whole will be better too, because health visiting must be seen to operate according to clear standards.

Using the grid to its correct extent, she considers the other layers. She feels that although Michael and Caroline's respective *autonomies* are *not being respected*, and that by not giving Michael a free hand in his private life *short-term autonomy is not being created*, everyone is being *respected equally* by the supervisor (no exceptions are being made), and *needs are being served first, before wants* (Michael wants to see Caroline but Caroline has no need – Michael's time could be better spent serving the needs of others).

Mary thinks about the red layer and concludes that the *truth is being told*, no *harm* is being done, and *positive good* is being produced – at least in the longer term. She carries out a similar analysis within the black layer, and her judgement remains the same. (Note that Mary seems not to have used the Grid to criticise her initial stance, but to support it. This is not always the best use of the Grid.)

## A Possible Use of the Grid by Dennis

Dennis does not start at the green layer, but with the blue core. His analysis goes like this.

He sets out to consider each blue box in turn, to see how it relates to the case in question. He begins with *create autonomy*, and decides there is no question that the autonomy of both Michael and Caroline is being impeded by the supervisor's decision. The requirement to *create autonomy by removing obstacles from people's physical and intellectual paths*, to enable them to take greater charge of their own destinies, is a foundational feature of health work. The question is: can the impairment of two people's autonomy be justified, either by pointing to greater future autonomy gain, or by showing that the beliefs and wishes of Michael and Caroline are somehow deficient, or both?

In this case the ideas of *creating* and *respecting* autonomy are not far apart. Unless their beliefs can be shown to be clearly mistaken it can hardly be denied that Michael and Caroline's choices are not being respected. As he considers the box *respect persons equally* it becomes clear to Dennis that this is the key consideration. He thinks that neither Michael nor Caroline are being afforded the basic respect due to persons. Caroline in particular is being abused. To use Kant's terminology, she is being used as a means rather than an end. She is not being treated as a person, but as an object. She has been used to train the health visitor. Her personal circumstances and needs are immaterial (indeed they always were to the supervisor), all that was necessary was that somebody was available to allow Michael to develop health visiting experience.

Dennis concludes that Michael is not being respected as a person either. All that seems to matter to the supervisor is that one more efficient, rule-following, functional health visitor has been trained, but Dennis is clear that work for health is not merely work against disease and illness, nor is it work only to create health in a patient (all who are part of an intervention should be considered). With this in mind he decides, provisionally, that the supervisor's action has offended against a vital principle. And, although he has only limited evidence, Dennis also judges it likely that Caroline does have needs which Michael can meet.

Having considered the blue layer, Dennis moves on to the other layers, prepared to reassess his provisional conclusions if necessary. He steps to the black level, the level of external considerations. What laws might come into play? Would the supervisor be legally able to punish Michael if he continued to see Caroline privately? This is unclear. Michael would certainly not be breaking any criminal or civil law, but the supervisor might attempt to initiate internal disciplinary procedures on the ground of 'unprofessional behaviour' – or some other charge she thinks might stick. Would such a course of action be likely? Can it be clearly established that Caroline does, in fact, have needs which justify health visitor support? Or is Michael being self-indulgent? What are the motives and goals of the three people involved? How genuine is Michael? All these matters, Dennis reviews.

After establishing as much as he can about the external circumstances, Dennis surveys the red and green levels, but does not spend too long on these (this time) because the blue core is primary, because the consequences are unpredictable, and whatever they might be, they will not be of significant import except to Michael, Caroline, and the supervisor.

Dennis finds that Michael should disobey the supervisor, explaining his reasons, and should continue with his mutually beneficial relationship. He selects the following boxes: *respect persons equally, maximise benefit for the individual* and *do most positive good.*

## ANALYSIS

Which of the two proposals is the most convincing? Which will produce the highest degree of morality?

Both health workers have deliberated with integrity. Both have used the Grid legitimately, yet they have produced conflicting responses.

A good case can be made out for both responses, however Dennis' position is more in tune with work for health, and suggests an approach that will increase morality to a higher degree. Of course, this cannot be demonstrated with certainty. As events unfold it might turn out that Mary's proposal would have been more satisfactory. But one can judge only on what seems likely at the time, on what evidence is available, and in accordance with whatever moral outlook one has chosen to live by. Because Dennis' proposal shows respect for the individuals involved, because it recommends a genuine attempt to directly enable those concerned (taking into account the likely outcomes in the long term), and because proper attention is paid to the potentials of the key actors rather than reference to some vague social good (it is not clear how this will be created by the supervisor's hard line – what difference to health visiting as a whole would her tough action really make?) Dennis' proposal appears to produce a higher degree of morality – in direct proportion to the enhancing potentials enabled in Michael and Caroline.

## 2.   SPONSORSHIP AND HIDDEN MOTIVES

Remember Professor Ronson, the Head of a Department of Community Medicine who wants the department to be involved in as many community research projects as possible, employing as many research staff as possible (pp. 60–61). The professor would like to embark on a research project to discover why there is a relatively low use of the medical and health facilities in one part of the city. The uptake rate is more or less what one would expect (fairly low because the area in question is the poorest in the district, with the highest levels of unemployment and single-parent families). However, the specific reasons are not known. Taking into account the fact that the local population suffers a disproportionately high level of disease and illness it seems important to understand more about why they act as they do.

Professor Ronson has exhausted his research budget, and has made it known to potential sponsors and research bodies that he wishes to undertake a two-year project, employing at least one research associate. Unfortunately for the professor, none of the usual sources of funds wishes or is able to help. Out of the blue there has been an offer of sponsorship from a famous tobacco company, which has told Professor Ronson it intends to fund worthwhile health research throughout the country and is pleased to say this is one of its first offers. The professor's dilemma is clear: should he accept sponsorship from a company which trades in a commodity which creates disease and illness?

Another way of expressing this question is to ask: what is the most ethical intervention the professor can make? Although there is no immediate intervention into other people's lives in this case, the repercussions of doing something or nothing are bound to affect others indirectly, and there might eventually be direct and dramatic effects.

## Two Contrasting Thoughts

### Claire's Thinking

Claire's immediate reaction is that Professor Ronson should not accept the tobacco company's money. To do so, she thinks, would be entirely unprincipled, would undermine the ethos of the health service, would reflect discredit on Professor Ronson, and would provide a valuable source of propaganda for the tobacco industry. The tobacco companies would, if their sponsorship were to be accepted, be able to claim they were being endorsed by the health service. Claire thinks that taking the money would be unquestionably wrong.

### Charlotte's Thinking

Even though Charlotte is aware that many people will feel there is something offensive about a sector of the health service accepting tobacco money, she does not regard this of crucial importance. She thinks about it, and sees there is much to be gained by accepting the sponsorship – many people may benefit if Professor Ronson takes the grant.

After all, Charlotte reflects, the health service is funded from a source that some consider more reprehensible than the tobacco companies. The state (or the government of the day) is by far the largest sponsor of the health service. And much of what the state does undoubtedly harms the health of the population (in a medical sense as well as in other senses). For instance, governments permit industrial pollution, manufacture nuclear weapons, allow people to suffer unemployment when, with alternative policies, they could ensure work for all. Yet very few researchers have any qualms about accepting funds from this source.

## THE USE OF THE GRID IN THIS CASE

It falls to each health worker to consider each level of the grid in some order, either to justify her initial thinking or to appreciate the merits of an alternative.

### Claire's Use of the Grid

Claire thinks that if Professor Ronson accepts the money then the balance of good over evil for society will be substantially decreased. Even if there is benefit for the professor, for the research associate, for the university, and for the disadvantaged section of the community in question, this will be outweighed by the increased credibility given to the tobacco companies.

Studying the red level she sees that there may be a duty incumbent on the professor to *minimise harm,* and she considers that to accept the offer will, indirectly, lead to harm. Claire is convinced the tobacco company's intent is not altruistic. It is seeking propaganda, and increasingly needs to show it can work for social good to help in its fight against measures to curtail its business. On considering the blue level, Claire reasons that the intervention is too indirect to raise issues of *autonomy, respect,* and *need.*

Claire thinks the professor should decline the sponsorship, and regards the boxes *minimise harm, and maximise benefit for society* of most significance.

## Charlotte's Use of the Grid

Charlotte also begins with the consequences layer, but remains of the view that the good consequences for the professor, the university, the disadvantaged group, and the research associate, outweigh the possible decrease in social good. After reflecting on the black layer Charlotte reasons that the effect on society is so open to speculation that the outcome of the professor's acceptance of sponsorship can be no more than a matter of opinion. It is just as likely that a fine research project could produce significant nationwide benefits for similar groups of people, and that direct and clear improvements in many people's life quality could result. There is no evidence that accepting the award would lead to more people smoking, nor is it certain that the tobacco company's efforts (whatever its motive) will do anything to prevent legislation against their marketing activities.

Charlotte considers that the box *do most positive good* is the most relevant on the red level, and also thinks the blue core important. She believes that a successful research project could lead to significant improvements in the autonomy of disadvantaged individuals, and will certainly enhance the scope and self-direction of the research associate, while even if there are spin-offs for the tobacco company these will not reduce general levels of autonomy.

In Charlotte's opinion Professor Ronson should accept the money, and denounce smoking at the same time if that is what he wishes. She regards the boxes *create autonomy, maximise benefit for self* and *maximise benefit for a particular group* of greatest significance.

## ANALYSIS

In my opinion, the appropriate analysis has already been carried out. For Charlotte's reasons, Professor Ronson should accept the money in order to create a higher degree of morality.

# TEN TIPS FOR TEACHING WITH THE ETHICAL GRID

The Ethical Grid is used widely to teach ethics to health professionals, but is not always employed to its full potential. To use the Grid most effectively a teacher should:

1. Introduce the Grid by *first* explaining its underpinning philosophy of health. Ideally the teacher should outline the foundations theory of health, and build up the four blue boxes as she does so (the handbook 'Suggestions and Guidance for Teachers and Lecturers', offered free with *Health Promotion: Philosophy, Prejudice and Practice*[5] provides extensive support in this regard). Once students have grasped the blue boxes' philosophical basis the teacher should add the Grid's outer layers one by one.
2. Allow students time to expose their initial thoughts and prejudices. Explain that the best use of the Grid is to challenge these biases – it is easy to use it unreflectively to confirm them, and this is a danger users should constantly appreciate.
3. Be clear that the best use of the Grid requires a very specific question or hypothesis.
4. Explain how the Grid works, using at least one real life example, before allowing students to work with it themselves.
5. Emphasise that it is the user, not the Grid, which does the analysing. This means that for each case the user must define afresh what each box means (what are the risks? what does benefit mean in this case? which harm should be minimised? and so on).
6. If using group work, appoint one member of the group as a neutral chairperson, to report back and to keep the others focused on the Grid. A neutral chairperson is also recommended if the Grid is used in teams and case conferences in actual cases.
7. Suggest that the chairperson takes notes of the deliberative process.
8. Note that it is best when first using the Grid to work systematically in, starting with the black layer and ending with the blue. Note too that once students have used the Grid this way a couple of times it is a good idea to ask them to 'home in' on any boxes which seem to 'stand out' for them, as they study the case at hand.
9. If teaching humanities or arts students point out that the Grid is a practical device. Though some of its terms may seem academically unsophisticated this is deliberate – challenge the students to solve practical problems firmly and confidently. If teaching practitioners point out that the Grid is derived from a long-standing academic tradition, and that all its categories are disputable. Allow this type of student to explore the black layer until she feels comfortable with the practical issues, then insist she pays attention to the more theoretical layers.
10. Deal with common misperceptions at the outset. For example:

    i. The Grid can produce conflicting responses to the same issue, but it cannot support *any* answer – at least one blue box should be used in keeping with the foundations theory of health.
    ii. The only relationships between the boxes are the colours. The combinations which make up the 'pyramid sides' are arbitrary.

iii. Grid users can select as many boxes as they wish, though three or less will normally be adequate. There is no obligation to select one of each colour. More than one of each colour can be chosen if desired.

iv. *Create autonomy* is most definitely not the same as *respect autonomy*.

## CONCLUSION

I hope that the Ethical Grid continues to be widely used. But more importantly I hope it is increasingly employed with knowledge of its philosophical background. I hope that as it is used in practice and teaching, more and more users understand that *all* work for health is a moral endeavour – not just bits of it. And as more health workers come to realise this truth – and commit to a substantial, well-articulated theory of health – I hope the new paradigm will finally gain sufficient power to eclipse the old one.

# References

1. Seedhouse, D. F. (1986). *Health: The Foundations for Achievement*, John Wiley, Chichester.
2. Gillon, R. (1985). *Philosophical Medical Ethics*, John Wiley, Chichester.
3. Beauchamp, T. and Childress, J. (1989). *Principles of Biomedical Ethics*, 3rd edition, Oxford University Press, New York and Oxford.
4. Johnstone, M.-J. (1994). *Bioethics: A Nursing Perspective*, Harcourt & Brace, Marrickville, NSW.
5. Seedhouse, D.F. (1997). *Health Promotion: Philosophy, Prejudice and Practice*, John Wiley, Chichester.
6. Parotid internet site – http://herston.uq.oz.au
7. Kent, G., Delany, L., Hope, T. and Grant, V. (independent authors – discussion forum) (1996). Teaching analysis. Informed consent: a case for multidisciplinary teaching. *Health Care Analysis* **4**(1), 65–79.
8. Proposal to establish a Bachelor of Health Science Degree, University of Auckland, 1997.
9. Seedhouse, D. F. (ed.) (1995). *Reforming Health Care: The Philosophy and Practice of International Health Reform*, John Wiley, Chichester.
10. Seedhouse, D. F. (1991). *Liberating Medicine*, John Wiley, Chichester.
11. West, R. and Trevelyan, J. E. (1985). *Alternative Medicine: A Bibliography of Books in English*, Mansell.
12. http://pespmc1.vub.ac.be/ASC/HOLISM.html
13. Greaves, D. (1979). What is medicine? Towards a philosophical approach. *Journal of Medical Ethics* **5**, 29–32.
14. Fulford, K. W. M. (1993). Bioethical blind spots: four flaws in the field of view of traditional bioethics. *Health Care Analysis* **1**(2), 155–162.
15. Metcalfe, D. (1989). Teaching communication skills to medical students. In, *Changing Ideas in Health Care*, ed. D. Seedhouse and A. Cribb, John Wiley, Chichester, pp. 219–230.
16. WHO (World Health Organisation) (1986). *Ottawa Charter for Health Promotion*, WHO.
17. Institute of Medical Ethics (1987). *Report of a Working Party on the Teaching of Medical Ethics* (The Pond Report), IME Publications, London.
18. Hébert, P. C., Meslia, E. M. and Dunn, E. V. (1992). Measuring the ethical sensitivity of medical students: a study at the University of Toronto. *Journal of Medical Ethics* **18**, 142–147.
19. Seedhouse, D. F. (1991). Against medical ethics: a philosopher's view. *Medical Education* **25**(4), 280–282.
20. United Kingdom Central Council for Nursing, Midwifery, and Health Visiting (1986). *Project 2000*.
21. Jackson, P. (1995). Processes of persuasion: social interests and total quality in a UK hospital trust. *Health Care Analysis* **3**(4), 283–289.
22. Holloway, F. (1996). Community psychiatric care: from libertarianism to coercion. Moral panic and mental health policy in Britain. *Health Care Analysis* **4**(3), 235–243.
23. Kuhn, T. S. (1970). *The Structure of Scientific Revolutions*, University of Chicago Press.
24. Kuhn, T. S. (1977). *The Essential Tension: Selected Studies in Scientific Tradition and Change*, University of Chicago Press.
25. Lakatos, I. and Musgrove, A. (1970). *Criticism and the Growth of Knowledge*, Cambridge University Press, Cambridge.
26. Wolf, F. A. (1981). *Taking the Quantum Leap*, Harper and Row, New York.
27. Ellis, W. D. (ed.) (1938). *A Source Book of Gestalt Psychology*, London.

28. Kenny, A. J. P. (1978). *Freewill and Responsibility*, Routledge and Kegan Paul, London.
29. Williams, A. (1995). Economics, QALYs and medical ethics – a health economist's perspective. *Health Care Analysis* **3**(3), 221–234.
30. Aristotle (1976). *Ethics*. Trans. by J. A. K. Thomson. Introduction by J. Barnes. Penguin edition, Harmondsworth.
31. Moore, G. E. (1903). *Principia Ethica*, Cambridge University Press, Cambridge, p. vii.
32. McKeown, T. (1979). *The Role of Medicine. Dream, Mirage or Nemesis?*, Blackwell, Oxford.
33. Rogers, A., Pilgrim, D., Gust, I., Stone, D. and Menzel, P. (independent authors – discussion forum) (1995). The pros and cons of immunisation. *Health Care Analysis* **3**(2), 99–107.
34. Brannigan, M. (1996). Designing ethicists. *Health Care Analysis* **4**(3), 206–218.
35. Britain's innocent addicts, *Observer*, 28 February 1988.
36. Thompson, E. P. (1985). The transforming power of the cross. In, *Religion and Ideology*, ed. R. Bocock and K. Thompson, Manchester University Press, Manchester.
37. Katch, F. I. and McArdle, W. D. (1983). *Nutrition, Weight Control and Exercise*, Lea and Febiger.
38. Seedhouse, D. F. (1994). AIDS, science and the totem. *Health Care Analysis* **2**(4), 273–278.
39. Flanagan, T. J. and Longmire, D. R. (1996). *Americans View Crime and Justice: A National Public Opinion Survey*, Sage Publications, Thousand Oaks, California.
40. BMA (1984). *The Handbook of Medical Ethics*, British Medical Association, London.
41. Society of Health Education Officers (1986). *Draft Code of Ethics*. Also see Greenberg-Gold, J. S. and Gold, R. S. (1977). *The Health Education Ethics Book*, McGraw-Hill, New York.
42. Warnock, G. J. (1971). *The Object of Morality*, Methuen, London.
43. Harris, J. (1985). *The Value of Life*, Routledge and Kegan Paul, London.
44. Locke, J. (1984). *An Essay Concerning Human Understanding*, Oxford University Press, Oxford.
45. Dewey, J. (1920). *Reconstruction in Philosophy* (1920, New York, New American Library, 1950).
46. Emmet, D. (1979). *The Moral Prism*, Macmillan, London.
47. Warnock, M. (1978). *Ethics Since 1900*, Oxford University Press, Oxford.
48. Kant, I. (1785). *Groundwork of the Metaphysics of Morals* (trans. H. J. Paton), Harper Torch Books edition, 1964.
49. Moore, G. E. (1903). *Principia Ethica*, Cambridge University Press, Cambridge.
50. Mill, J. S. (1910). *Utilitarianism, Liberty and Representative Government*, Dent edition, London.
51. Raphael, D. D. (1981). *Moral Philosophy*, Oxford University Press, Oxford.
52. Beauchamp, T. and Childress, J. (1979). *Principles of Biomedical Ethics*, 1st edition, Oxford University Press, New York and Oxford.
53. Beauchamp, T. L. (1994). The 'four principles' approach. In, *Principles of Health Care Ethics*, ed. R. Gillon, John Wiley, Chichester.
54. Gillon, R. (ed.) (1994). *Principles of Health Care Ethics*, John Wiley, Chichester.
55. Miller, D. (1976). *Social Justice*, Clarendon Press, Oxford.
56. Rawls, J. (1973). *A Theory of Justice*, Oxford University Press, Oxford.
57. Seedhouse, D. F. (1994). *Fortress NHS: A Philosophical Review of the National Health Service*, John Wiley, Chichester.
58. Seedhouse, D. F. (1995). The way around health economics' dead end. *Health Care Analysis* **3**(3), 205–220.
59. Seedhouse, D. F. (1997). What's the difference between health care ethics, medical ethics and nursing ethics? *Health Care Analysis* **5**(4), 267–274.
60. Seedhouse, D. F. (1997). The inescapable prejudice of health economics: a reply to Farrar, Donaldson, Macphee, Walker and Mapp. *Health Care Analysis* **5**(4), 310–314.
61. Williams, A. (1985). The value of QALYs. *Health and Social Science Journal* **94**(4967) (18 July), 3–4 of Supplement (following p. 904).
62. *The Economist*, 10 January 1987.
63. Mooney, G., Gerard, K., Donaldson, C. and Farrar, S. (1992). *Priority Setting in Purchasing: Some Practical Guidelines*, National Association of Health Authorities and Trusts, Birmingham, UK.
64. Palmer, G. (1996). Casemix funding of hospitals: objectives and objections. *Health Care Analysis* **4**(3), 185–193.
65. Koestler, A. (1978). *Janus: A Summing Up*, Hutchinson, London.
66. *Hansard*. House of Lords, 10 November 1987, cols 1350–1351.

67. *Bolam* v *Friern Hospital Management Committee* [1957] 2 All ER 118 [1957] 1 WLR 582.
68. Harrison, B. (1979). *An Introduction to the Philosophy of Language*, Macmillan, London.
69. World Health Organisation (1980). *Mental Disorders: Glossary and Guide to their Classification in Accordance with the Ninth Revision of the International Classification of Diseases*, WHO, Geneva.
70. Koestler, A. and Smythies, J. R. (1972). *Beyond Reductionism, New Perspectives in the Life Sciences*, Hutchinson, London.
71. *Gillick* v *West Norfolk and Wisbeck Area Health Authority* [1984] 1 All ER 365 per Woolf J; revsd [1985] 1 All ER 533, CA; revsd [1985] 3 All ER 402, HL.
72. DHSS Guidelines (H C (86) 1), HMSO, London.
73. Brazier, M. (1987). *Medicine, Patients and the Law*, Penguin, Harmondsworth.
74. *R* v *Arthur* (1981).
75. *Re B (a minor)* [1981] 1 WLR 1421.
76. Nowell-Smith, P. (1994). In favour of voluntary euthanasia. In, *Principles of Health Care Ethics*, ed. R. Gillon, John Wiley, Chichester.
77. Beauchamp, T. L. and McGullough, L. (1984). *Medical Ethics*, Prentice-Hall, Englewood Cliffs, NJ.
78. Seedhouse, D. F. and Cribb, A. (1989). *Changing Ideas in Health Care*, John Wiley, Chichester.
79. Baum, M., Zilkha, K. and Houghton, J. (1989). Ethics of clinical research: lessons for the future. *British Medical Journal* **299**, 251–253.
80. Christie, R., Freer, C., Hoffmaster, C. B. and Stewart, M. A. (1989). Ethical decision making by British general practitioners. *Journal of the Royal College of General Practitioners* **39**, 448–451.
81. Waldron, J. (ed.) (1984). *Theories of Rights*, Oxford University Press, Oxford.
82. Baum, M. (1988) I didn't abuse my patients. *Observer*, 16 October, p. 8.
83. *Guardian*, 4 December 1988.
84. *Guardian*, 9 December 1988.
85. Seedhouse, D. F. and Lovett, L. (1992). *Practical Medical Ethics*, John Wiley, Chichester.

# Index

Note: page numbers in *italics* refer to figures

ability to do  184
act-deontology  115–16
  disadvantages  116
act-utilitarianism  125–6, 127
acting morally  122
  Kant's theory  118–20
actions
  ethical content  7
  justification by reference to evidence  208
acts, judgement of
  illegal and amoral 92,  *93*
  illegal and immoral  92, *93*
  illegal and moral  92, *93*
  legal and amoral  92, *93*
  legal and immoral  91, *93*
  legal and moral  91, *93*
aesthetic pleasure  43
ailing paradigm  101
alternative medicine  24
apartheid  143
Aristotle  44, 120
arrest, arbitrary  133
autonomy
  ability to do  184
  consent  186, 187, 189–91
  consideration of  191
  creation  179–80, 182, 183, 185, 186, 220
    autonomy flip  192, 193
    removing obstacles  215
    respect persons equally  202
  devaluation  181
  diminishing  195, 197, 199
  drug abuse  183
  encouraging maximum  86, 87
  enhancing  183
  flip  98, 183, 192–3, 196, 201
    drug abuse  193
  health care  180–1
  human quality  184–6

importance  191
  increasing  195, 197, 198, 199
  laws  182
  mental  194, 196, 197
  mental handicap/illness  185, 187
  physical  194, 196, 197
  as a quality  182-3
  ranking ideas with  192–3
  respect for  128, 182, 185, 202, 220
    autonomy flip  192, 193
    removing obstacles  215
  richness  181–3
  as a right  181–2
  single principle  181
  test  150, 194–8
    applying  198–9
    limitations  199–203
    unwanted  137
awareness  7–8
Ayer, A. J.  94

bad faith  135–8
  throwing off  137–8
Beauchamp, Tom  128, 129, 130, 131
behaviour principles, Kant's view  117
being ethical  52
beneficence  128
Bentham, Jeremy  124, 141
bioethics  45, 128
biological potential  102
Bryant, Martyn  128
businessperson (case study)  71

capital punishment  88
caregiving (case study)  71
caring (case study)  56–7
case conferences  211–12
categorical imperative  118–19, 121
  interpretation  121

certainty
    moving away from   150, 151
    moving closer to   150
Childress, Jim   128, 129, 130, 131
choice
    future   107
    respect for   191
choosing, independent   137
citizens, enablement   109
clinical trials, consent   188–91
clinician role   24
Clouser, K. D.   129, 130
codes of practice, professional   89, 90–1, 208
coercion (case study)   63–4
communication
    effects of news   158–9
    Rings of Uncertainty   149, 157–60
    shock   159–60
communication between doctors and
        patients   24
community
    members   119, 120
    moral   120
Community Medicine professor (case study)
        60–1, 216–18
competence see technical competence
comprehension   158
conduct of life deliberations   39–40
confidence, information holding   86–7
confusions, ethical   205
consent
    autonomy   186, 187, 188–91
    clinical trials   188–91
    for operation   156
consequences
    Ethical Grid   218
    ethics   123–4
    green layer   205–6
    Kant's views   117, 123
    moral philosophy   43
    motive   123
    rule-utilitarianism   128
consequentialism   123–4, 205
    QALYs   141
contraceptive advice   160–2
contracts, legally enforceable   91
cost-benefit calculation, utilitarianism   124
course of action   xiv
criminals, Kant's views   123
crisis period, paradigm change   29
cultural norms   94
cultural relativism   96
culture
    political   110
    values dependent on   80

death, truth   64

decision-making   149
decisions, injustice   143
defensive medicine/nursing   155
deliberation
    ethics   145
    personal   137
    process   44–5
    health workers   47
democracy, British   138
democratic society   109
deontology   43, 114–17
    Ethical Grid red layer   205
    types   115–17
Dewey, John   109–10
dialysis
    ranking of potential beneficiaries   206
    rationing   66
discrimination, QALYs   142, 143
disease
    medical work   55
    prevention   32
district nurse (case study)   63–4
divine law   117
doctor–nurse relationship (case study)   69
dramatic ethics   38, 39, 40, 41
drawing lots   144
drug abuse
    autonomy   183
    autonomy flip   193
drug education (case study)   65
drug supply for volunteers (case study)   70–1
duty
    abiding by pure motive   122
    hierarchy   114
    Kant's ethics   117
    moral person   114
    moral philosophy   43
    single overriding   114
    see also deontology
dwarfing   xiv, 11
    deliberate   100
    gratuitous   204
    health work against   100–3
    immorality   111
    ranking   201
    selective   107
dying (case study)   171–5

economic inequality   133
economists, injustice of QALYs   141, 142
education
    egalitarian   134
    ethics   24
    nursing   24
egotism   95–6, 121
emotional needs, detection   51
emotivism   94–5

empowering 31
enablement 101, 204
　citizens 109
　physical 51
　potentials 110
essence 136
ethical A 7, 8, *9*
ethical B 7–8, *9*
ethical confusions 205
ethical content 7
Ethical Grid xiv, 2–4, 11, 209
　act-deontology 115
　analogy 177–9
　ascertainment of wishes 208
　autonomy creation 202
　black layer 207-8
　blue layer 179–204
　circular version *5*
　classic theories of Western moral philo-
　　sophy 114
　consequences 218
　creating autonomy 179–81, 182, 183, 185,
　　186, 192, 193
　designing 3–4
　dimensions 178
　enhancement of deliberation 208–9
　ethics B 8
　external considerations 207
　green layer 205–6
　group work 219
　health worker case 214–16
　hypothesis 211
　justification of actions by reference to
　　evidence 208
　law 207–8
　layers 177, 178
　limits 209
　misperceptions 219–20
　moral reasoning 209, 212
　practice 211
　prescriptive ethical theory 120
　red layer 204–5
　Rings of Uncertainty 153, 165, 171
　specific questions 211
　teaching with 219–20
　use 11–12, 177–8, 211–18
ethical intervention 104
ethical principles 180
ethical realm 8, *9*
ethical template 2–4
ethical theory
　moral maxim consideration 87
　moral reasoning 113–14
ethical thinking 113–14
ethics
　actions 7
　assessment xiii

conflicts 37
　of consequences 123–4
　education 24
　everyday 36, 37
　in a general sense 38, 39–40, 41
　　values 78–9
　health work xiii
　health workers 45
　inconsistencies 36
　key importance 47–8
　law distinction 91–2, *93*
　nature of 2
　objective 85–7
　Rings of Uncertainty 160–2
　statements 97
　teaching 1–2
　　tools 3
　training 24
　work for health 35–6
　*see also* dramatic ethics; everyday ethics;
　　persisting ethics; technical ethics
euthanasia 88
　non-voluntary 143
evangelicism 85
everyday ethics 36, 37
exercise advice
　undesirable consequences 82
　values 81–4
existence 137
　valuing 106

facts 97
　moral theory foundation 98
fairness 131, 141
　justice as 132–4
faith, shared 117
Falklands conflict 40
Felicific Calculus 141
fitness definition 82
foundations theory of health 184, 186
four principles approach to medical ethics
　128–31
full human being 106
　*see also* humans

games, rules 88–90
gender 143
general practitioner performing minor opera-
　tion 163–4
general utilitarianism 126
Gert B 129, 130
gestalt trauma 33
gestalt-switch 29–30, 31
gestalt-trap 32
Gillick, Victoria 85, 161
Gillick case 160
Gillon, Raanan 129, 130, 131

goodness
  aesthetic pleasure  43
  moral  43
  nature of  42–3
  useful objects  42
group work, Ethical Grid  219
growth
  mental 101
  as only true moral end 109–10
  physical  101

handicapped infants  143
  case study  167–71
harm
  in health care  86
  minimising  121, 218
  moral outcome  128
Harris, John  105, 106-7, 108, 144
health
  disease reference  32–3
  ethics  107
  theories of  5–6, 7
health care
  autonomy  179–81
  changes  xii
  crisis  28–9
  decisions  149–50
  defining by medicine  23
  harm  86
  hierarchical organisation  11
  human interest  123
  intellectual crisis  33, 45
  landmarks  23–4
  orthodox  1
  paradigm change  27, 29, 33
  paradigm shift  xii, 9–10
  political aspect  110
  purpose  23
  right to (case study)  73
  values  23
health creation  51–2
  ethical commitment  35
health economists, view of ethics  35
health education officer (case study)  57–8, 65
health educators  33
health funds, cost-effective use  140
health interventions  48–50
  choices  51
  moral calibre  50
  nature  52
  types  52–3
health management  10
health professionals, codes of practice  89,
    90–1
health promotion  32
health service  10
  assumptions  204

enablement of citizens  109
injustice of decisions  143
interventions in the name of health  203–4
moral concern  134
providing basic needs  202
rationing  66
health visitor
  case study  56–7, 59–60, 212–14
  value permeation of work  82–4
health work  xi
  against dwarfing  100–3
  aims  6
  breadth  102
  conceptual developments  25
  current practice  55
  ethics  8
  existing rationale  204
  future choice  107
  limits in Rings of Uncertainty  162
  moral endeavour  xiii
  moral obligations  205
  moral work  34
  morality link  47–50
  nature  47
  theoretical limits  6
  values  81–4
  see also work for health
health workers
  choice of actions  49
  discovery of potentials  108
  education in moral reasoning  144–5
  encouraging maximum autonomy  86, 87
  ethics  45
  future change through present practice  31
  Kant's ethical theory  122–3
  key question  47, 50–1
  legal accountability  90
  paradigm change  33–4
  promotion of way of thinking  114
  rule-utilitarianism  127
  rules  90
heart attack, potential  157
Hitler, A.  143
holistic medicine  24, 29
honesty, true feelings  86
human activity, meaning of  xi
human condition, shared  203
human flourishing  44
human interest  123
human morality, value relationship  80
human potential  107
  abstract terms  107
  deliberate restriction  110–11
  empirical investigation  108
  enablement  110
  enhancement  44
  enhancing latent  198

prohibiting 107
specific 108
human rights 182
humans
  moral importance 98
  morality 103
  *see also* full human being

iceberg
  representation of ethics 8, 9
  tip 38–42
ideal state creation 100
ideas, ranking with autonomy 192–3
ideologies, values 79
illness, medical work 55
immorality 99–100
  dwarfing 111
  restriction of individual potential 110–11
  selective dwarfing 107
immunisation
  case study 59–60
  education 126
inequality 133
  justice 132
intellectual crisis 45
intellectual potential 102
introspection, discovering laws 122
irrational world 135
irrationality 94

judgement, personal 150
justice 128, 131–4
  contractual 132
  as fairness 131–4, 141
  inequality 132
  social 133

Kant, Immanuel 117–23
kindness 123
knowledge, Aristotle's divisions 44
Kuhn, Thomas 25, 27, 29, 30

language 157, 158
law
  autonomy 182
  discovering 122
  divine 117
  Ethical Grid 207–8
  impartial system 133
  morality conflict 91
  morality distinction 91–2, 93
  Rings of Uncertainty 155–7, 161–2
lawful behaviour 91
legal rights 182
legislation, moral 90–2, 93
liberties, basic 133

liberty
  Kantian ethics 120
  rights to 133
life circumstances, dealing with unexpected 137
living thing, valuable 106
Locke, John 105

medical school curriculum (case study) 72
medical services 10
medical treatment, wartime 203
medical work, ethics 107
mental handicap, autonomy 185, 187
mental illness 41–2
  autonomy 185, 187
  case study 67–8
mental patient
  abandonment 143
  autonomy 185, 187
  sterilisation 199–201
military defence 143, 144
Moore, G. E. 124
moral code, binding 87–90
moral endeavour
  nature 47
  *see also* work for health is a moral endeavour
moral evangelists 85
moral intervention xiii–xiv
moral legislation 90–2, 93
moral maxims, apparently objective 87
moral philosophy
  consequences 43
  deliberation process 44–5
  duties 43
  understanding good 42–3
moral reasoning 80, 113–14
  education for medical practitioners/health workers 144–5
  Ethical Grid 209, 212
  explicit 212
  obstacles 135–45, 145
  transcending given rules 138
moral reflection, subjective opinion 95
moral rules, breaking 88
moral work 34
morality *see* ethics
morphine overprescription (case study) 69
mother, dying (case study) 171–2
motives
  consequences 123
  moral path 122
  pure 118, 122
murder 88

National Health Service (NHS) 10
needs, serving 202–3
Newtonian mechanics, paradigm shift 25–6
non-intervention, radical 52

non-maleficence   128
nurse
    education   24
    practice   155–7
    Rings of Uncertainty   151–3
nurse practitioner's dilemma (case study)   62
nurse–doctor relationship (case study)   69

objective morality   85–7
objectivism   93–4
objects, distinctions from people   136
obligations, consideration   205
obstacle elimination   47
opportunism   125

paid work, values   80
pain, language   157
painkiller overprescription (case study)   69
Paradigm X   26, 27, 28
paradigm change   xiv
    case studies   55
    crisis period   29
    health care   27, 29, 33
    health workers   33–4
    Kuhn's theory   25, 26, 27
    process   11
    through present practice   31
    transition   31
paradigm shift   xii
    abstract   27
    health care   9–10
    Newtonian mechanics   25–6
Paradigm Y   9, 10, 11, 18, 19
    autonomy test   194
    formation   30
    impetus   28
    policy-makers   28
    successor to Paradigm X   26, 27
parenting   99
paternalism   192, 196
perception
    Behaviourist account   29–30
    Gestalt school   29, 30
persisting ethics   38, 39, 40
person
    basic sense   53
    definition   105
    distinctions from objects   136
    ends in themselves   118, 119
    equality of basic characteristics   111
    full   53
    meaning   53
    as means   191
    needs   132
    principle of equal respect   106, 202
    rational   133–4
    treatment as ends   123

true to self   115
truly moral   118
personal deliberation   137
personal judgement, rule-utilitarianism   126
personal maturity   113
personhood   xiv, 204
    characteristics   111
    criteria   106, 108
philosophy of health/medicine   xi
physical potential   102
political culture   110
political liberty   133
politics, Kant's theory   120
positive health   31
potential
    development   102
    enhancing   204
principles
    moral   80
    values   79
priorities in health care   140
problem-solving, options   151
professional codes of practice   89, 90–1, 208
professionals
    act-deontology   115–16
    moral obligation   86
    predefined role   135
promises
    breaking   120, 122
    deceitful   122
    keeping   91, 121
property ownership rights   132, 133
punishment, appropriate   131

QALYs   139–45
    arbitrary content   142
    benefit   143–4, 145
    criteria   142
    discrimination   142, 143
    injustice   141–2, 143
    myth promotion   142–3
    subjective value imposition   142
    treatment outcomes   142
    use   140–1
Quality Adjusted Life Years see QALYs

race   143
rationalist   133–4
rationing health services   66
Rawls, John   132–4
reality
    losing touch   135
    Rings of Uncertainty   151
reason, acting morally   122
reasoned wishes, overriding   198
reasoning see moral reasoning
reflection, discovering laws   122

relativism 93, 94
  cultural 96
  types 94–6
religious justification 117
repression 182
resources
  equal distribution 133
  plus technical competence 153–5
  Rings of Uncertainty 153–5
  *see also* scarce resources
respect
  autonomy 128, 192, 193
  principle of equal 106
responsibility, individual 125
rights, autonomy as 181–2
Rings of Uncertainty 149
  case studies 167–75
  communication 157–60
  Ethical Grid 153, 165, 171
  ethics 160–2
  fully expressed *158*
  key dictum 164–5
  law 155–7, 161–2
  limits of health work 162
  quantification 165, 167
  reality 151
  relative importance of considerations 165,
    *166*
  resources 153–5
  scoring 165, 167
  steps
    one 150–2
    two 151–3
    three 162
    four 163–4
    five 164–5
    six 165, *166*
  technical competence 151–3, 155
  tensions 157
rule-deontology 116–17
rule-followers, committed 137–8
rule-utilitarianism 126–8
  moral outcome from harm 128
rules
  benefits 90
  conforming 90
  God-given 117
  health work ethics 90
  legitimate 88–90
  pregiven 138
  training to habitually follow 137

Sartre, Jean-Paul 135, 136
scarce resources
  distribution 122, 141, 144
  public knowledge 145
Seedhouse, D. 98

self-consciousness 106
self-indulgence 215
self-interest 119
  pursuit 95
  sacrifice 124
shock, communication 159–60
slavery 119–20
social choices 137
social inequality 133
social institutions 109
social justice 133
social work, parenting 99
society
  cultural relativism 96
  democratic 109
  immorality 99–100
specific ethics *see* dramatic ethics
sponsorship (case study) 60–1, 216–18
  ethical intervention 217
statements of fact/morality 97
sterilisation, mental patient 199–201
subjective opinion 95

team meetings 212
technical competence
  plus resources 153–5
  Rings of Uncertainty 151–3, 155
technical ethics 36, 37–8, 42–5
  deliberation process 44–5
  moral maxim consideration 87
  nature of goodness 42–3
teleological ethics 114
terminally ill people, care 108
tragic choice 39
  case study 61–2
  public recording 145
training, ethics 24
transplant organs, resources 154–5
treatment
  assessment 140
  costs 140
  outcomes 142
  selection for 141
true nature 135
truth
  absolute 86
  death 64
  standards 94
  telling 121, 126, 127
  case study 57–8

uncertainty, communication 159
universal standards, relativism 96
universalisability 123
utilitarian ethics 114
utilitarianism 43, 123, 124
  cost-benefit calculation 124

utilitarianism (*continued*)
　goals　124
　green layer　205–6
　types　125–8

value conflicts　77–8
　resolving　85–98
value judgement　xiii, 84
　emotivism　94, 95
values
　aesthetic　78, 79
　cultural　80
　distinguishing　78
　ethical implications　78–9
　evangelicism　85
　exercise advice　81–4
　health visitor work permeation　82–4
　health work　81–4
　human morality relationship　80
　ideologies　79
　innate　80
　intangible　78, 79
　paid work　80
　principles　79
　types　78
　ultimate/ultimate ordering　85–7
　variety　84
valuing
　own existence　106
　subjects within a culture　80
　types　79

vision defects　101–2

Warnock, Mary　106, 108
wartime, medical treatment　203
welfare　192, 193
Western moral philosophy　114
Williams, Alan　139
work for health　6
　ethics　35–6
　eye checks for children　101
　foundation role　101
　full person creation　108
　intervention types　48
　meaning　32
　moral commitment　7
　needs of people　132
　practical　108
　removal of obstacles to people's biological/
　　intellectual potentials　204
　*see also* health work
work for health is a moral endeavour　xiii, 6,
　8, 10, 35–6
　biological potential　98
　human potential　98
　routine interventions　50
World Health Organisation (WHO), ideal
　state　179
wrist, broken　48–51

*Index compiled by Jill Halliday*